Michael Schulte-Markwort / Kath (.)

Cross-walks: ICD-10 –

MW01131631

Michael Schulte-Markwort
Kathrin Marutt
Peter Riedesser
(Editors)

Cross-walks: ICD-10 – DSM IV-TR

A Synopsis of Classifications of Mental Disorders

With Forewords by Horst Dilling and Hans-Ulrich Wittchen

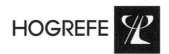

Library of Congress Cataloging-in-Publication Data
is now available via the Library of Congress Marc Database under the
LC Control Number 2003104138

National Library of Canada Cataloging-in-Publication Data

Cross-walks: ICD 10 - DSM IV-TR : a synopsis of classifications of mental disorders / Michael Schulte-Markwort, Kathrin Marutt, Peter Riedesser (eds.).

Includes bibliographical references.
ISBN 0-88937-268-3

1. Mental illness—Diagnosis. 2. Mental illness—Classification. 3. Diagnosis, Differential. 4. International statistical classification of diseases and related health problems. 5. Diagnostic and statistical manual of mental disorders.
I. Schulte-Markwort, Michael II. Marutt, Kathrin III. Riedesser, Peter

RC455.2.C4C76 2003   616.89'075   C2003-901950-0

Second printing 2008
Copyright © 2003, 2008 by Hogrefe & Huber Publishers

PUBLISHING OFFICES
USA: Hogrefe & Huber Publishers, 875 Massachusetts Avenue, 7th Floor,
                Cambridge, MA 02139,
                Phone (866) 823-4726, Fax (617) 354-6875, E-mail info@hogrefe.com
Europe: Hogrefe & Huber Publishers, Rohnsweg 25, D-37085 Göttingen, Germany,
                Phone +49 551 49609-0, Fax +49 551 49609-88, E-mail hh@hogrefe.com

SALES & DISTRIBUTION
USA: Hogrefe & Huber Publishers, Customer Service Department,
                30 Amberwood Parkway, Ashland, OH 44805,
                Phone (800) 228-3749, Fax (419) 281-6883, E-mail custserv@hogrefe.com
Europe: Hogrefe & Huber Publishers, Rohnsweg 25, D-37085 Göttingen, Germany,
                Phone +49 551 49609-0, Fax +49 551 49609-88, E-mail hh@hogrefe.com

OTHER OFFICES
Canada: Hogrefe & Huber Publishers, 1543 Bayview Avenue, Toronto, Ontario, M4P 3B5
Switzerland: Hogrefe & Huber Publishers, Länggass-Strasse 76, CH-3000 Bern 9

Hogrefe & Huber Publishers
Incorporated and Registered in the State of Washington, USA, and in Göttingen, Lower Saxony, Germany

Printed and bound in the USA
ISBN 978-0-88937-268-9

Forewords

In 1993, H.-J. Freyberger and E. Schulte-Markwort and I published the reference tables for the German version of ICD-9/ICD-10 Chapter V. Our work, which was published as part of a series called *Fortschritte der Psychiatrie und Neurologie [Progress in Psychiatry and Neurology]*, was still incomplete at that time because appropriate tables allowing for "conversions" between ICD-10 and DSM-IV were still lacking. Now, M. Schulte-Markwort, K. Marutt and P. Riedesser have prepared these *Cross-walks*, which is basically an annotated commentary on the classifications, based on ICD-10 and DSM-IV-TR. Numerous notes and comparison tables show where the two classifications differ –for instance, time criteria. Users can see at a glance which disorders are missing from each classification, or where the correspondence between the two is not 100%. At the same time, it is equally easy to identify where there are significant differences between ICD-10 and DSM-IV diagnoses, despite the same term being used. However, it also becomes clear that the majority of diagnoses can be readily transferred from one classification to the other – a welcome contrast to the vast differences that existed between ICD-9 and ICD-10.

This comparative closeness between the international and American classifications gives me some hope that a global classification will be available one day. I wish this book, which is ideally suited for practical use, the success it deserves among those working in adult as well as child and adolescent psychiatry.

Lübeck, Germany, May 2003

Horst Dilling

Forewords

"What? Yet another book on the classification of mental disorders! To make matters worse, one on a topic that should have been clarified by the DSM-IV Manual, with its ICD-10-compatible codes, and by the various ICD-10 material books." This or similar reactions to the cross-walk book of Schulte-Markwort, Marutt, and Riedesser might be expected from those physicians who take the view that the field of mental disorder classification has finally come to rest.

As understandable as this reaction may be at first sight, the wish for an extended "time out" concerning our handling of diagnostic criteria that is expressed thereby is highly dangerous:

The classification of mental disorders and behavioral disturbances is and will remain an ongoing challenge, given the abundance of new neurobiological, neuropsychological, and epidemiological findings and advances that continue to emerge. These advances mean that we must continually reconsider our paradigms, and in particular re-examine our diagnostic "habits" and classifications and revise them if necessary. Diagnostic classification will always remain the central link between basic or applied research and clinical practice. Therefore, we can not allow idiosyncratic habits to develop on the basis of uncritical diagnostic classification, as often happened in the past. In the end, such habits will rapidly start to interfere once again with the diagnostic "communication" that we have worked so hard to improve over recent years, and will thus also interfere with scientific progress and, ultimately, patient welfare.

In view of this, this book of cross-walks is a valuable and practical resource, in the first place for colleagues in research and science. The complex distinctions and differences between ICD-10 and DSM-IV-TR are dealt with in a clear, appropriate, and differentiated manner, providing outstanding guidance for a more careful, critical and appropriate handling of diagnostic classification. At the same time, the cross-walks show on closer inspection how far away we still are from the goal of a globally recognized, uniform diagnostic classification system.

Personally, I believe such a goal is highly desirable but not immediately imperative, because I cannot see how such a globally uniform system could ever be sensibly implemented to the same extent in, for instance, developing countries with their relatively basic health system and highly industrialized areas with their highly differentiated and specialized care services. Similar doubts might be voiced with regard to the differing requirements of ophthalmologists, psychotherapists, and neurobiological researchers.

In any event, this book of cross-walks is without doubt an excellent support tool for all those planning research projects, whether this be in the basic or in the clinical field. In addition, it will both make a definite contribution towards a better handling of diagnostic classification systems, and at the same time encourage suggestions for appropriate revisions of the ICD and the DSM-IV classifications.

Dresden/Munich, Germany, May 2003

Hans-Ulrich Wittchen

Introduction

ICD-10 (WHO, 1992) and DSM-IV-TR (APA, 1994, 2000) are the two internationally established diagnostic manuals for mental disorders during adulthood as well as childhood and adolescence. Following a period of transition from the old manuals ICD-9 and DSM-III(-R), which was accompanied by various publications and cross-walks (for instance Cooper, 1988; Thompson & Pincus, 1989; Freyberger, Schulte-Markwort, & Dilling, 1993a, 1993b; Remschmidt & Schmidt, 1994), both new systems have now become broadly accepted and established. The predominantly held opinion is that the similarities between ICD-10 and DSM-IV are stronger than those between each classification and its respective predecessor (Pitzer & Schmidt, 2000). On closer inspection, however, it becomes apparent that there are sometimes significant differences, with comparatively little research on their consequences (First & Pincus, 1999). The American literature generally seems to proceed on the assumption that DSM-IV represents a "de facto standard" or has rule character (Maser et al., 1991, First & Pincus, 1999) while ICD-10, being the "European system" (First & Pincus, 1999), follows specific traditions of European psychiatry and has more of a guideline character (Thangavelu & Martin, 1995). This applies, for example, to the differences in the conception of the schizo-affective and some of the affective disorders. Further differences exist without any real rationale and have repeatedly been criticized as ethnocentric (Alarcon, 1995). The danger of ignoring phenomenological, intersubjective, and inherently historical key concepts in classification systems was pointed out by Jablensky (1999).

There is a structural difference between ICD-10 and DSM-IV in that ICD-10 additionally defines research criteria (WHO, 1993: Dilling et al., 1994) whilst these only appear in DSM-IV as supplementary diagnoses described in the appendix. An important paradigmatic difference consists in the requirement of the DSM-IV that the patient concerned has to be restricted by the symptoms, whereas this criterion does not appear in ICD-10. The DSM-IV system generally follows more psychopathologic principles, while the chapters of ICD-10 are structured pathogenetically. In order to develop a sensible and practical cross-walk, one therefore has to proceed in both directions, coming from both ICD-10 and DSM-IV. So far, one cross-walk was published by van Drimmelen-Krabbe, Bertelsen and Pull (1999) and another with a special focus on child and adolescent psychiatric diagnoses by Pitzer and Schmidt (2000). The numerous publications dealing with diagnosis-specific differences cannot be considered here as they would be beyond the scope of this manual.

The possibility of coding co-morbid diagnoses is specific to ICD-10's child and adolescent psychiatric diagnoses and not available in this form in DSM-IV.

Multiaxial diagnosis within adult psychiatry is still at an early stage. While child and adolescent psychiatry has been diagnosing multiaxially since 1975 (Rutter et al.) and proceeds hexaxially today (Remschmidt & Schmidt, 1994), DSM-IV only provides for the possibility of multiaxial diagnosis without there being any agreement on its being binding (Saß, Wittchen and Zaudig, 1998).

The correspondence between ICD-10 and DSM-IV varies from 33% (criteria for disorders caused by abuse of psychotropic substances) to 87% (for dysthymia). The average correspondence is 68% (Andrews, Slade, &Peters, 1999). These figures demonstrate how necessary and appropriate a cross-walk is that allows readers quick access to the correspondences and differences. Even if Saß, Wittchen and Zaudig are of the opinion that "the two classifications ICD-10 and DSM-IV appear to be different dialects of the same language," the emphasis on the correspondence between the two systems and on efforts at bringing them closer together (especially within the last decade) must not obscure the fact that sometimes different dialects are hard to understand. The differences also protect us from the danger of relying too easily on the supposed invariability of psychiatric classification systems, in clinical as well as research contexts, without fulfilling the essential function of thinking about improvements and adjustments (Kendell, 1991). A diagnosis can only be fully understood in the combination of syndromal diagnosis and nosologic factors (Bertelsen, 1999).

The tables presented here include all updates contained in DSM-IV-TR and are intended for clinical use as well as for research purposes. They are meant to help avoid complicated comparisons of the two manuals by listing the most important differences under the heading "cross-walk." Mere differences in phrasing or a specific choice of words are not taken into account as they would have necessitated printing both classifications in their entirety next to each other, which would have considerably lessened the practical usefulness of the book. This manual is not meant to replace or stifle scientific debate on the comparisons between ICD-10 and DSM-IV-TR, or indeed an adjustment of the classifications. Pitzer and Schmidt have good reason to warn of the "danger of superficial simplification of psychiatric matters instead of fully utiliz-

ing differentiated classification possibilities" due to an uncritical use of reference tables.

The present manual thus intends to Purpo

- Provide an overview of the comparability
- Represent a working basis for a faster translation of codings and
- Offer a basis for continuing research.

We hope that we can thereby contribute a little towards a continuing constructive globalization within the field of psychiatry and psychotherapy as well as child and adolescent psychiatry and psychotherapy. In this, we agree with H. Dilling (1998), who expressed his hope for a globally recognized system for the classification of mental disorders.

Like all publications of this kind, this cross-walk depends on the feedback of its readers. We would be especially grateful for indications of any mistakes — which we have of course striven to avoid!

Our special thanks go to Prof. H. Dilling and Prof. H.-U. Wittchen who did not hesitate to place their forewords in front of the manual.

Hamburg, Germany, May 2003

Michael Schulte-Markwort,
Katrin Marutt,
Peter Riedesser

Directions for Use of the Tables

The left-hand column of the first table lists all ICD-10 diagnoses of chapter V (mental disorders) according to the clinical-diagnostic guidelines. The right-hand column gives the matching diagnoses under DSM-IV-TR.

The second table presents the reverse relation. The left-hand column lists the diagnoses according to DSM-IV-TR. The corresponding ICD-10 diagnoses can be found in the right-hand column.

Whenever the classification system on the right does not provide for the diagnosis given on the left, instructions as to how to code the disorder are given in italics. Only in a few instances is it impossible to give definite coding instructions without additional information; this is marked accordingly.

For a quick overview, the column "cross-walk" contains information on the correspondence between the two systems of diagnosis, indicated by arrows:

⟷ A double arrow indicates complete correspondence.

⟵ An arrow pointing to the left indicates that this diagnosis or differentiation is only provided for in this system.

Significant differences in the diagnostic criteria between ICD-10 and DSM-IV-TR, in spite of otherwise matching diagnoses (e.g., statements on symptom duration), are pointed out in the cross-walk.

DSM-IV-TR allows for further differentiation of various diagnoses without separate coding. The respective references can also be found in the cross-walk.

Whenever additional codings or differentiations are stated at the beginning of a chapter, they apply to all diagnoses within that chapter. Otherwise they appear directly with the respective diagnosis. The indenting of the diagnoses and additional differentiations in the respective columns provides for an easy and quick overview of the matches.

Note
The last part of the second table (DSM-IV-TR – ICD-10) contains the section on "other clinically relevant problems." In this chapter, the correspondence relations are mostly based on the information given in DSM-IV-TR as far as **non-psychiatric** diagnoses are concerned. These are included in the table for completeness' sake; however, the correspondence relations have not been examined further. This can be seen from the lack of entries in the cross-walk column.

ICD-10 – DSM-IV-TR

	ICD-10	cross-walk		DSM-IV-TR
F0	**Organic, Including Symptomatic, Mental Disorders**			**Delirium, Dementia, Amnestic and Other Cognitive Disorders**
	F0x.x0 Without additional symptoms F0x.x1 With additional symptoms, predominantly delusional F0x.x2 With additional symptoms, predominantly hallucinatory F0x.x3 With additional symptoms, predominantly depressive F0x.x4 Other mixed symptoms	Codes on the 5th character of the ICD-10 for F00 to F03. The corresponding categories of the DSM can be found in the respective sections. Duration of the disorder ≥ 6 months in the ICD-10, no time periods given in the DSM.		
F00	**Dementia in Alzheimer's Disease**		294.10 294.11	**Dementia of the Alzheimer's Type** ... Without Behavioral Disturbance ... With Behavioral Disturbance
F00.0	With early onset	←——→		With Early Onset
F00.1	With late onset	←——→		With Late Onset *Differentiation in the DSM without separate code. In case it is impossible to definitely classify as 294.10 or 294.11, code as 294.8 Dementia NOS.*
F00.2	Atypical or mixed type	←—		*In case it is impossible to definitely classify as 294.10 or 294.11 code as 294.8 Dementia NOS.*
F00.9	Unspecified	←—		
F01	**Vascular Dementia**	←——→	290.4	**Vascular Dementia**
F01.0	Vascular dementia of acute onset	*No directly corresponding categories in the DSM.*		Vascular Dementia...
F01.1	Multi-infarct dementia			
F01.2	Subcortical vascular dementia			
F01.3	Mixed (cortical and subcortical) vascular dementia	←—	290.4 290.41 290.42 290.43	Uncomplicated With Delirium With Delusions With Depressed Mood
F01.8	Other vascular dementia	Cf. 5th character of the ICD-10 or F05 Delirium		
F01.9	Vascular dementia, unspecified			

	ICD-10	cross-walk		DSM-IV-TR
F02	**Dementia in Other Diseases Classified Elsewhere**			**Dementia Due to Other General Medical Conditions**
F02.0	Dementia in Pick's disease	⟷	294.10	Dementia Due to Pick's disease
F02.1	Dementia in Creutzfeldt-Jakob disease	⟷	294.10	Dementia Due to Creutzfeldt-Jakob Disease
F02.2	Dementia in Huntington's disease	⟷	294.1	Dementia Due to Huntington's Disease
F02.3	Dementia in Parkinson's disease	⟷	294.1	Dementia Due to Parkinson's Disease
F02.4	Dementia in human immunodeficiency virus (HIV) disease	⟷	294.9	Dementia Due to HIV Disease
F02.8	Dementia in other specified diseases classified elsewhere	⟷	294.1	Dementia Due to ... [Indicate the General Medical Condition]
F03	**Unspecified Dementia**	⟷	**294.8**	**Dementia NOS**
F04	**Organic Amnesic Syndrome, Not Induced by Alcohol and Other Psychoactive Substances**	⟷	**294.0**	**Amnestic Disorder Due to a General Medical Condition**
F05	**Delirium, Not Induced By Alcohol and Other Psychoactive Substances**			**Delirium Due to a General Medical Condition**
F05.0	Delirium, not superimposed on dementia	⟷	293.0	Delirium Due to ... *Cf. above (F00 and F01)*
F05.1	Delirium, superimposed on dementia	⟷ ⟷	290.11 / 290.3 / 290.41	
F05.8	Other delirium	⟷	293.0	Delirium Due to ...
F05.9	Delirium, unspecified	⟷	780.09	Delirium NOS
F06	**Other Mental Disorders Due to Brain Damage and Dysfunction and to Physical Disease**			**Psychotic Disorders Due to a General Medical Condition**
F06.0	Organic hallucinosis	⟷	293.82	Psychotic Disorders Due to ... With Hallucinations
F06.1	Organic catatonic disorder	⟷	293.89	Catatonic Disorder Due to ...
F06.2	Organic delusional (schizophrenia-like) disorder	⟷	293.81	Psychotic Disorder Due to... With Delusions
F06.3	Organic mood (affective) disorders	⟷	293.83	Mood Disorder Due to ...
F06.30	Organic manic disorder	⟷		With Manic Features
F06.31	Organic bipolar disorder	⟵		*No corresponding differentiation.*

	ICD-10	cross-walk		DSM-IV-TR
F06	**Other Mental Disorders Due to Brain Damage and Dysfunction and to Physical Disease**	**Continuation**		**Mental Disorders Due to a General Medical Condition**
F06.32	Organic depressive disorder	←——→ Classification in the DSM depends on whether or not all the criteria for Major Depression Episode are fulfilled.		With Major Depression-Like Episode With Depressed Features
F06.33	Organic mixed affective disorder	←——→		With Mixed Features
F06.4	Organic anxiety disorder	←——→	293.84	Anxiety Disorder Due to ...
F06.5	Organic dissociative disorder			
F06.6	Organic emotionally labile (asthenic) disorder			*No corresponding category for F06. to F06.8, code as 294.9 Cognitive Disorder NOS.*
F06.7	Mild cognitive disorder			* For F06.7 cf. Appendix B – Mild Neurocognitive Disorder.*
F06.70 F06.71	Nonorganic Organic	←—		*For F06.8 possibly also codes for Sexual Dysfunction or Sleep Disorder Due to a General Medical Condition, see below.*
F06.8	Other specified mental disorders due to brain damage and dysfunction and to physical disease			
F06.9	Unspecified mental disorders due to brain damage and dysfunction and to physical disease	←——→	239.9	Psychotic Disorder NOS Due to ...
F07	**Personality and Behavioral Disorders Due to Brain Disease, Damage and Dysfunction**	←——→	310.1	**Personality Change Due to a General Medical Condition**
F07.0	Organic personality disorder			*No corresponding category, code as 310.1 Personality Change Due to ... * **[Indicate the General Medical Condition]** *.*
F07.1	Postencephalitic syndrome			* For F07.1 and F07.2 maybe also 294.9 Cognitive Disorder NOS.*
F07.2	Postconcussional syndrome			* For F07.2 cf. Appendix B – Postconcussional Disorder.*
F07.8	Other organic personality and behavioral disorders due to brain disease, damage and dysfunction	←—		
F07.9	Unspecified organic personality and behavioral disorders due to brain disease, damage and dysfunction			
F09	**Unspecified Organic or Symptomatic Mental Disorder**		293.9	**Mental Disorder NOS Due to ...**

	ICD-10	cross-walk		DSM-IV-TR
F1	**Mental and Behavioral Disorders Due to Psychoactive Substance Use**			**Substance-Related Disorders**
	F10 Disorders due to use of alcohol F11 Disorders due to use of opioids F12 Disorders due to use of cannabinoids F13 Disorders due to use of sedatives or hypnotics F14 Disorders due to use of cocaine F15 Disorders due to use of other stimulants, including caffeine F16 Disorders due to use of hallucinogens F17 Disorders due to use of tobacco F18 Disorders due to use of volatile solvents F19 Disorders due to multiple drug use and use of other psychoactive substances	Codes on the 3rd character of ICD-10 for classification of substances. For classification of substances under DSM refer to the respective diagnoses. (Code phencyclidine under F19 in ICD-10).		
F1x.0	Acute Intoxication ...	⟷ Classification of substances in ICD-10 see above.	303.0 292.89 305.90	... Intoxication Alcohol Amphetamine, Cannabis, Hallucinogen, Inhalants, Cocaine, Opioid, Phencyclidine, Sedative, Hypnotic or Anxiolytic, Other (or Unknown) Substance Caffeine
F1x.00	Uncomplicated			
F1x.01	With trauma or other bodily injury	⟵		*No corresponding differentiation.*
F1x.02	With other medical complications			
F1x.04	With perceptual distortions	⟷		... With Perceptual Disturbances
F1x.05	With coma			
F1x.06	With convulsions	⟵		*No corresponding differentiation.*
F1x.07	Pathological intoxication			
F1x.03	With delirium	⟷ Classification of substances in ICD-10 see above.	291.0 292.81	... Intoxication Delirium Alcohol Amphetamine, Cannabis, Hallucinogen, Inhalants, Cocaine, Opioid, Phencyclidine, Sedative, Hypnotic or Anxiolytic, Other (or Unknown) Substance

	ICD-10	cross-walk		DSM-IV-TR
F1x.1	Harmful use	←→ Classification of substances in ICD-10 see above.	305.x	... Abuse 00 – Alcohol ; 70 – Amphetamine; 20 – Cannabis; 90 – Hallucinogen ; 90 – Inhalant ; 60 – Cocaine; 50 – Opioid ; 90 – Phencyclidine ; 90 – Sedative, Hypnotic or Anxiolytic ; 90 – Other (or Unknown) Substance
F1x.2	Dependence syndrome	←→ Symptoms ≥ 1month in the ICD-10 or repeatedly within 12 months. No duration given in the DMS for an observation period of 12 months. Classification of substances in ICD-10 see above.	303.90 304.x	... Dependence Alcohol 40 – Amphetamine ; 30 – Cannabis ; 50 – Hallucinogen ; 60 – Inhalant ; 20 – Cocaine; 10 – Nicotine ; 00 – Opiate ; 90 – Phencyclidine ; 10 – Sedative, Hypnotic or Anxiolytic ; 90 – Other (or Unknown) Substance
F1x.20	Currently abstinent *No directly corresponding category*	← All additional differentiation in the DSM for substance dependence without separate codes.		*No directly corresponding category.* Early Full Remission Early Partial Remission Sustained Full Remission Sustained Partial Remission
F1x.21	Currently abstinent, but in a protected environment	←→		In a Controlled Environment
F1x.22	Currently on a clinically supervised maintenance or replacement regime	←→		On Agonist Therapy
F1x.23	Currently abstinent, but receiving treatment with aversive or blocking drugs	←		*No corresponding differentiation.*
F1x.24	Currently using the substance	←		
F1x.25	Continuous use	←		*No corresponding differentiation.*
F1x.26	Episodic use (dipsomania)	←		
F1x.3	Withdrawal state	←→	291.81 292.0	... Withdrawal Alcohol Amphetamine, Cocaine, Nicotine, Opiate, Sedative, Hypnotic, or Anxiolytic Other (or Unknown) Substance
F1x.30	Uncomplicated	←		*No corresponding differentiation.*
F1x.31	With convulsions	←		*No corresponding differentiation.*

	ICD-10	cross-walk		DSM-IV-TR
F1x.4	Withdrawal state with delirium	◄——► Classification of the substances in the ICD-10 see above.	291.0 292.81 292.81	... Withdrawal Delirium Alcohol - Sedative, Hypnotic, or Anxiolytic Other (or Unknown) Substance
F1x.40	Uncomplicated	◄——		*No corresponding differentiation.*
F1x.41	With convulsions	◄——		*No corresponding differentiation.*
F1x.5	Psychotic disorder ...			Psychotic or Mood Disorder
F1x.50	Schizophrenia-like	◄——		*No corresponding category, code as 291.9 or 292.9 (cf. F1x.9).*
F1x.51	Predominantly delusional	◄——► Classification of the substances in the ICD-10 see above.	291.5 292.11	... Psychotic Disorder with Delusions Alcohol-Induced Persisting Amphetamine-, Cannabis-, Hallucinogen-, Inhalant-, Cocaine-, Opioid-, Phencyclidine-, Sedative-, Hypnotic-, or Anxiolytic-Induced, Other (or Unknown) Substance-Induced
F1x.52	Predominantly hallucinatory	◄——► Classification of the substances in the ICD-10 see above.	291.3 292.12	... Psychotic Disorder With Hallucinations Alcohol-Induced Persisting Amphetamine-, Cannabis-, Hallucinogen-, Inhalant-, Cocaine-, Opioid-, Phencyclidine-, Sedative-, Hypnotic-, or Anxiolytic-Induced Other (or Unknown) Substance-Induced
F1x.53	Predominantly polymorphic	◄——		*No corresponding category, code as 291.9 or 292.9 (cf. F1x.9).*
F1x.5	Psychotic disorder ...	Classification of substances in ICD-10 see above. Additional differentiation in the DSM without separate codes.	291.89 292.84	Psychotic or Mood Disorder ... Mood Disorder Alcohol-Induced Amphetamine-, Hallucinogen-, Inhalant-, Cocaine-, Opioid-, Phencyclidine-, Sedative-, Hypnotic-, or Anxiolytic-Induced Other (or Unknown) Substance-Induced
F1x.54	Predominantly depressive symptoms	◄——►		With Depressed Features
F1x.55	Predominantly manic symptoms	◄——►		With Manic Features
F1x.56	Mixed	◄——►		With Mixed Features
F1x.6	Amnesic syndrome	◄——► Classification of substances in ICD-10 see above.	291.1 292.83	... Persisting Amnestic Disorder Alcohol-Induced Inhalant-, Sedative-, Hypnotic-, or Anxiolytic-Induced Other (or Unknown) Substance-Induced

	ICD-10	cross-walk		DSM-IV-TR
F1x.7	Residual and late-onset psychotic disorder			
F1x.70	Flashbacks	←——→	292.89	Hallucinogen Persisting Perception Disorder (flashback)
F1x.71	Personality or behavior disorder	←——		*No corresponding category, code as 291.9 or 292.9 (cf. F1x.9).*
F1x.72	Residual affective disorder			
F1x.73	Dementia	←——→		... Persisting Dementia
		Classification of substances in ICD-10 see above.	291.2	Alcohol-Induced
			292.82	Inhalant-, Sedative-, Hypnotic-, or Anxiolytic-Induced
				Other (or Unknown) Substance-Induced
F1x.74	Other persisting cognitive impairment			
F1x.75	Late-onset psychotic disorder	←——		*No corresponding category, code as 291.9 or 292.9 (cf. F1x.9).*
F1x.8	Other mental and behavioral disorders			
F1x.9	Unspecified mental and behavioral disorder	←——→		... -Related Disorder NOS
		Classification of substances in ICD-10 see above.	291.9	Alcohol
			292.9	Amphetamine-, Cannabis-, Hallucinogen-, Inhalant-, Caffeine-, Cocaine-, Nicotine-, Opioid-, Phencyclidine-, Sedative-, Hypnotic-, or Anxiolytic-, Other (or Unknown) Substance
F2	**Schizophrenia, Schizotypal and Delusional Disorders**			**Schizophrenia and Other Psychotic Disorders**
		The 5th character of the ICD-10 encodes onset patterns. Differentiation without separate code in the DSM.		
F20.x0	Continuous	←——→		Continuous
F20.x1	Episodic with progressive deficit	←———————→		Episodic With Interepisode Residual Symptoms
F20.x2	Episodic with stable deficit	←—		
F20.x3	Episodic remittent	←——→		Episodic With No Interepisode Residual Symptoms
F20.x4	Incomplete remission	←——→		Single Episode, In Full Remission
F20.x5	Complete remission	←——→		Single Episode, In Partial Remission

	ICD-10	cross-walk		DSM-IV-TR
F2	**Schizophrenia, Schizotypal and Delusional Disorders**	**Continuation**		**Schizophrenia and Other Psychotic Disorders**
	F20.x8 Other	←——→		Other or Unspecified Pattern
	F20.x9 Period of observation < 1 year	←——		*No corresponding category.*
F20	**Schizophrenia**	Observation period ≥ 6 months in the DSM.		**Schizophrenia**
F20.0	Paranoid schizophrenia	←——→	295.30	Paranoid Type
F20.1	Hephrenic schizophrenia	←——→	295.10	Disorganized Type
F20.2	Catatonic schizophrenia	←——→	295.20	Catatonic Type
		In ICD-10 symptoms ≥ 2 weeks.		
F20.3	Undifferentiated schizophrenia	←——→	295.90	Undifferentiated Type
F20.4	Post-schizophrenic depression	←——		*No corresponding category, code as 298.9 Psychotic Disorder NOS.* *(Cf. Appendix B – Postpsychotic Depressive Disorder of Schizophrenia)*
F20.5	Residual schizophrenia	←——→	295.60	Residual Type
F20.6	Simple schizophrenia	This Diagnosis in the ICD-10 is not recommended to be made.		*No corresponding category, code as 298.9 Psychotic Disorder NOS.* *(Cf. Appendix B – Simple Deteriorative Disorder)*
F20.8	Other Schizophrenia	←——		*No corresponding category, code as 298.9 Psychotic Disorder NOS.*
F20.9	Schizophrenia, unspecified			
F21	**Schizotypal Disorder**	←——		*No directly corresponding category, code most likely as 301.22 Schizotypal Personality Disorder, otherwise as 298.9 Psychotic Disorder NOS.*
F22	**Persistent Delusional Disorders**			**(Schizophrenia and ...) Other Psychotic Disorders**
F22.0	Delusional disorder	←——→	297.1	Delusional Disorder
		Symptoms >3 months in the ICD-10, in the DSM >1 month. Respective disorders of <3 months are coded under F23 in the ICD-10.		
F22.8	Other persistent delusional disorder	←——		*No corresponding category, code as 297.1.*
F22.9	Persistent delusional disorder, unspecified	←——		*No corresponding category, code as 297.1.*

	ICD-10	cross-walk		DSM-IV-TR
F23	**Acute and Transient Psychotic Disorders**	← → Symptoms < 3 months in the ICD-10, for F23.1 and F23.2 < 1 month (for differentiation from F20 Schizophrenia). Symptoms are generally < 1 month in the DSM, otherwise code as 297.1.	**298.8**	**Brief Psychotic Disorder**
	F23.x0 Without associated acute stress F23.x1 With associated acute stress	Codes on the 5th character of the ICD-10. No separate codes for the subtypes in the DSM.		Without Marked Stressor(s) With Marked Stressor(s)
F23.0	Acute polymorphic psychotic disorder without symptoms of schizophrenia			
F23.1	Acute polymorphic psychotic disorder with symptoms of schizophrenia			
F23.2	Acute schizophrenia-like disorder	←		*No corresponding differentiation.*
F23.3	Other acute predominantly delusional psychotic disorder			
F23.8	Other acute and transient psychotic disorders			
F23.9	Acute and transient psychotic disorders, unspecified			
F24	**Induced Delusional Disorder**	← →	**297.3**	**Shared Psychotic Disorder**
F25	**Schizoaffective Disorders**	← → Additional differentiation in the DSM without separate codes.	**295.70**	**Schizoaffective Disorder**
F25.0	Schizoaffective disorder, manic type	← →		Bipolar Type (Manic Episode)
F25.1	Schizoaffective disorder, depressive type	← →		Depressed Type
		Criteria for F25.0 and F25.1 are widely spread in the ICD-10, therefore there are partially overlaps with 296.x4. Consider criteria!		*Possibly code also as 296.x4 Affective Disorder With Psychotic Features.*
F25.2	Schizoaffective disorder, mixed type	← →		Bipolar Type (Mixed Episode)
F25.8	Other schizoaffective disorders	←		*No corresponding differentiation.*
F25.9	Schizoaffective disorder, unspecified			

	ICD-10	cross-walk		DSM-IV-TR
F28	Other Nonorganic Psychotic Disorders	←		*No corresponding category, code as 298.9 Psychotic Disorder NOS.*
F29	Unspecified Nonorganic Psychosis	←→	298.9	Psychotic Disorder NOS
F3	Mood (Affective) Disorders			Mood Disorders
F30	Manic Episode			Manic Episode
F30.0	Hypomania	← *Without separate code in the DSM, Only able to be coded as part of a Bipolar II Disorder.*		*Code most likely as 296.89 Bipolar II Disorder (Hypomanic Episode).* *Also consider 296.80 Bipolar Disorder NOS.*
F30.1	Mania without psychotic symptoms	←→		Bipolar I Disorder, Single Manic Episode ...
F30.2	Mania with psychotic symptoms	←→	296.04	Severe With Psychotic Features
F30.20	... With mood-congruent psychotic symptoms	←→		Mood-Congruent Psychotic Features
F30.21	... With mood-incongruent psychotic symptoms	←→ *Differentiation without separate codes in the DSM.*		Mood-Incongruent Psychotic Features
F30.8	Other manic episodes	←		*No corresponding category, code as 296.80 Bipolar Disorder NOS.*
F30.9	Manic, episode, unspecified			
F31	Bipolar Affective Disorder			Bipolar Disorders
	F31.xx0 Only depressive episodes (not for F31.3, F31.4 and F31.5) F31.xx1 Only hypomanic or manic episodes F31.xx2 Only mixed episodes F31.xx3 Hypomanic, manic, depressive and/ or mixed episodes	← *More precise classification of the episodes that occurred during the anamnesis on the 6th character of the ICD-10.*		*No corresponding differentiation.*
F31.0	Bipolar affective disorder, current episode hypomanic	←→	296.40	Bipolar I Disorder, Most Recent Episode Hypomanic
	Bipolar affective disorder, current episode manic			Bipolar I Disorder, Most Recent Episode Manic ...
F31.1	... Without psychotic symptoms	← → → →	296.41 296.42 296.43	Mild Without Psychotic Features Moderate Without Psychotic Features Severe Without Psychotic Features *If the severity is not definitely attributable, code most likely as 296.80 Bipolar Disorder NOS.*

	ICD-10		cross-walk			DSM-IV-TR
F31	**Bipolar Affective Disorder**		**Continuation**			**Bipolar Disorders**
F31.2	... With psychotic symptoms		←→		296.44	Severe With Psychotic Features
F31.20	... Mood-congruent		←→			Mood-Congruent Psychotic Features
F31.21	... Mood-incongruent		←→			Mood-Incongruent Psychotic Features
			Differentiation without separate codes in the DSM.			
	Bipolar affective disorder, current episode ... depression					Bipolar I Disorder, Most Recent Episode Depressed ...
F31.3	... Mild or moderate ...		← →		296.51	Mild Without Psychotic Features
			→		296.52	Moderate Without Psychotic Features
F31.30	... Without somatic syndrome					*No corresponding differentiation.*
F31.31	... With somatic syndrome					
F31.4	... Severe ... ... Without psychotic symptoms		←→		296.53	Severe Without Psychotic Features
F31.5	... Severe ... ... With psychotic symptoms		←→		296.54	Severe With Psychotic Features
F31.50	... Mood-congruent		←→			Mood-Congruent Psychotic Features
F31.51	... Mood-incongruent		←→			Mood-Incongruent Psychotic Features
			Differentiation without separate codes in the DSM.			
F31.6	Bipolar affective disorder ... Current episode mixed		←→		296.6	Bipolar I Disorder, Most Recent Episode Mixed...
F31.7	Bipolar affective disorder, currently in remission		←			*No corresponding category, code under the various Bipolar Disorders in the DSM-IV-TR (Additional code In Full/Partial Remission), otherwise as 296.8 Bipolar Disorder NOS.*
F31.8	Other bipolar affective disorder		← ←→			*No corresponding category, code as 296.80 Bipolar Disorder NOS.*
F31.9	Bipolar affective disorder, unspecified		←→		296.80	Bipolar Disorder NOS
F32	**Depressive Episodes**		←→			**Major Depression, Single Episode**
F32.0	Mild depressive episode		←		296.21	Mild
F32.00	Without somatic syndrome					*No corresponding differentiation.*
F32.01	With somatic syndrome					

	ICD-10		cross-walk		DSM-IV-TR
F32	**Depressive Episodes**		**Continuation**		**Major Depression, Single Episode**
F32.1	Moderate depressive episode		←——→	296.22	Moderate
F32.10	Without somatic syndrome		←——		*No corresponding differentiation.*
F32.11	With somatic syndrome				
F32.2	Severe depressive episode ... Without psychotic symptoms		←——→	296.23	Severe ... Without Psychotic Features
F32.3	... With psychotic symptoms		←——→	296.24	... With Psychotic Features
F32.8	Other depressive episodes		←——		*No corresponding category, code as 311 Depressive Disorder NOS.*
F32.9	Depressive episode, unspecified		←——→	311	Depressive Disorder NOS
F33	**Recurrent Depressive Disorders**				**Major Depression, Recurrent**
F33.0	Current episode mild		←——→	296.31	Mild
F33.00	Without somatic syndrome		←——		*No corresponding differentiation.*
F33.01	With somatic syndrome		←——→		
F33.1	Current episode moderate			296.32	Moderate
F33.10	Without somatic syndrome		←——		*No corresponding differentiation.*
F33.11	With somatic syndrome				
F33.2	Current episode severe ... Without psychotic symptoms		←——→	296.33	Severe ... Without Psychotic Features
F33.3	... With psychotic symptoms		←——→	296.34	... With Psychotic Features
F33.4	Currently in remission		←—— ——→ ——→	296.35 296.36	In Partial Remission In Full Remission
					If not definitely attributable, code as 296.3
F33.8	Other recurrent depressive disorders		←——		*No corresponding category, code as 311 Depressive Disorder NOS.*
F33.9	Recurrent depressive disorder, unspecified		←——→		*No directly corresponding category, code as 311 Depressive Disorder NOS.*
F34	**Persistent Mood (Affective) Disorders**				
F34.0	Cyclothymia		←——→	301.13	Cyclothymic Disorder
F34.1	Dysthymia		←——→	300.4	Dysthymic Disorder
F34.8	Other persistent mood (affective) disorders		←——		*No corresponding category, code as 296.90 Mood Disorder NOS.*
F34.9	Persistent mood (affective) disorder, unspecified				

	ICD-10	cross-walk		DSM-IV-TR
F38	**Other Mood (Affective) Disorders**			
F38.0	Other single mood (affective) disorders			
F38.00	Mixed affective episode			
F38.1	Other recurrent mood (affective) disorders	←		*No corresponding category, code as 296.90 Mood Disorder NOS.*
F38.10	Recurrent brief depressive disorder			
F38.8	Other specified mood (affective) disorders			
F39	**Unspecified mood affective disorder**	←→	**296.90**	**Mood Disorder NOS**
F4	**Neurotic, Stress-Related and Somatoform Disorders**			**Anxiety Disorders, Somatoform Disorders**
F40	**Phobic Anxiety Disorders**			
F40.0	Agoraphobia ...			
F40.00	Without panic disorder	←→	300.22	Agoraphobia Without History of Panic Disorder
F40.01	With panic disorder	←→	300.21	Panic Disorder With Agoraphobia
F40.1	Social phobias	←→	300.23	Social Phobia
F40.2	Specific (isolated) phobias	←→	300.29	Specific Phobia
F40.8	Other phobic anxiety disorders	←		*No corresponding category, code as 300.00 Anxiety Disorder NOS*
F40.9	Phobic anxiety disorder, unspecified	←		*No directly corresponding category, code as 300.00 Anxiety Disorder NOS.*
F41	**Other Anxiety Disorders**			
F41.0	Panic disorder (episodic paroxysmal anxiety)	←→	300.01	Panic Disorder Without Agoraphobia
F41.1	Generalized anxiety disorder	←→	300.02	Generalized Anxiety Disorder
F41.2	Mixed anxiety and depressive disorder			*No corresponding category, code as 300.00 Anxiety Disorder NOS.*
F41.3	Other mixed anxiety disorders	←		*For F41.2 cf. Appendix B – Mixed Anxiety-Depressive Disorder.*
F41.8	Other specified anxiety disorders			
F41.9	Anxiety disorder, unspecified	←→	300.00	Anxiety Disorder NOS.

	ICD-10	cross-walk		DSM-IV-TR
F42	**Obsessive-Compulsive Disorder**		**300.3**	**Obsessive-Compulsive Disorder**
F42.0	Predominantly obsessional thoughts or ruminations			
F42.1	Predominantly compulsive acts (obsessional rituals)			
F42.2	Mixed obsessional thoughts and acts	←		*No corresponding differentiation, code as 300.3 Obsessive-Compulsive Disorder.*
F42.8	Other obsessive-compulsive disorders			
F42.9	Obsessive-compulsive disorder, unspecified			
F43	**Reaction to Severe Stress, and Adjustment Disorders**			
F43.0	Acute stress reaction	←→ Onset < 1 hour after the stress factor, subsiding after 8-48 hours in the ICD-10. No time periods given in the DSM.	308.3	Acute Stress Disorder
F43.1	Post-traumatic stress disorder	←→ Minimum period 1 month in the DSM.	309.81	Posttraumatic Stress Disorder
F43.2	Adjustment disorders ...			Adjustment Disorder ...
F43.20	Brief depressive reaction (<1 month)	← ←→	309.0	With Depressed Mood
F43.21	Prolonged depressive reaction (< 2 years)	←		
F43.22	Mixed anxiety and depressive reaction	←→		*No corresponding category, code as 309.9 Adjustment Disorder Unspecified.*
F43.23	With predominant disturbance of other emotions	←	309.28	With Mixed Anxiety and Depressed Mood
F43.24	With predominant disturbance of conduct	←→	309.3	With Disturbance of Conduct
F43.25	With mixed disturbance of emotions and conduct	←→	309.4	With Mixed Disturbance of Emotions and Conduct
F43.28	With other specified predominant symptoms	←		*No corresponding category, code as 309.9 Adjustment Disorder Unspecified.*
F43.8	Other reaction to severe stress			
F43.9	Reaction to severe stress, unspecified	←→	309.9	Adjustment Disorder Unspecified

	ICD-10	cross-walk		DSM-IV-TR
F44	**Dissociative (Conversion) Disorders**			**Conversion Disorder**
F44.0	Dissociative amnesia	←→	300.12	Dissociative Amnesia
F44.1	Dissociative fugue	←→	300.13	Dissociative Fugue
F44.2	Dissociative stupor	←		*No corresponding category, code as 300.15 Dissociative Disorder NOS.*
F44.3	Trance and possession disorders			*For F44.3 cf. Appendix B – Dissociative Trance Disorder.*
F44.4	Dissociative motor disorders	←→	300.11	... With Motor Symptom or Deficit
F44.5	Dissociative convulsions	←→	300.11	... With Seizures or Convulsions
F44.6	Dissociative anaesthesia and sensory loss	←→	300.11	... With Sensory Symptom or Deficit
F44.7	Mixed dissociative (conversion) disorders	←→	300.11	... With Mixed Presentation
F44.8	Other dissociative (conversion) disorders			
F44.80	Ganser's syndrome	←		*No corresponding category, code as 300.15 Dissociative Disorder NOS.*
F44.81	Multiple personality disorder	←→	300.14	Dissociative Identity Disorder
F44.82	Transient dissociative (conversion) disorders occurring in childhood and adolescence	←		*No corresponding category, code as 300.15 Dissociative Disorder NOS.*
F44.88	Other specified dissociative (conversion) disorders			
F44.9	Dissociative (conversion) disorder, unspecified	←→	300.15	Dissociative Disorder NOS
F45	**Somatoform Disorders**			**Somatoform Disorders**
F45.0	Somatization disorder	←→ Symptoms ≥ 2 years in the ICD-10, "several years" in the DSM.	300.81	Somatization Disorder
F45.1	Undifferentiated somatoform disorder	←→	300.82	Undifferentiated Somatoform Disorder
F45.2	Hypochondriacal disorder	←→	300.7	Hypochondriasis
F45.3	Somatoform autonomic dysfunction			
F45.30	Heart and cardiovascular system			
F45.31	Upper gastrointestinal tract			
F45.32	Lower gastrointestinal tract	←		*No corresponding category, code as 300.15 Dissociative Disorder NOS.*
F45.33	Respiratory system			
F45.34	Genitourinary system			
F45.38	Other organ or systems			

	ICD-10		cross-walk			DSM-IV-TR	
F45	**Somatoform Disorders**		**Continuation**			**Somatoform Disorders**	
F45.4	Persistent somatoform pain disorder (≥ 6 months) *(If necessary, code the additional illness)*		← → →		307.80 307.89	Pain Disorder Associated With Psychological Factors *Disorder Associated With Both Psychological Factors and a General Medical Condition*	
F45.8	Other somatoform disorders		←			*No corresponding category, code as 300.81 Somatoform Disorder NOS*	
F45.9	Somatoform disorder, unspecified		← →		300.82	Somatoform Disorder NOS	
F48	**Other Neurotic Disorders**						
F48.0	Neurasthenia		←			*No corresponding category, code as 300.82 Somatoform Disorder NOS.*	
F48.1	Depersonalization-derealization syndrome		← → ←		300.6	Depersonalization Disorder	
F48.8	Other specified neurotic disorders					*No corresponding category, code most likely as 300.9 Unspecified Mental Disorder (nonpsychotic).*	
F48.9	Somatoform disorder, unspecified						
F5	**Behavioral Syndromes Associated With Physiological Disturbances and Physical Factors**						
F50	**Eating Disorders**					**Eating Disorders**	
F50.0	Anorexia nervosa		← →		307.1	Anorexia Nervosa,	
F50.00	... Without active measures for loss of weight (Vomiting, Laxatives, etc.)		← →			Restrictive Type	
F50.01	... With active measures for loss of weight (Vomiting, Laxatives, etc.)		← →			"Binge-Eating/Purging"-Type	
F50.1	Atypical anorexia nervosa		← It is not recommended to make this diagnose in the ICD-10.			*No corresponding category, code as 307.50 Eating Disorder NOS.*	
F50.2	Bulimia nervosa		← →		307.51	Bulimia Nervosa	
F50.3	Atypical bulimia nervosa		← It is not recommended to make this diagnose in the ICD-10.			*No corresponding category, code as 307.50 Eating Disorder NOS.*	

	ICD-10	cross-walk		DSM-IV-TR
F50	**Eating Disorders**	**Continuation**		**Eating Disorders**
F50.4	Overeating associated with othe psychological disturbances			
F50.5	Vomiting associated with other psychological disturbances	←		*No corresponding category, code as 307.50 Eating Disorder NOS*
F50.8	Others, including: psychogenic loss of appetite			
F50.9	Eating disorder, unspecified		307.50	Eating Disorder NOS
F51	**Nonorganic Sleep Disorders**			**Sleep Disorders**
F51.0	Nonorganic Insomnia	←→	307.42	Primary Insomnia
F51.1	Nonorganic Hypersomnia	←→	307.44	Primary Hypersomnia
F51.2	Nonorganic disorder of the sleep-wake schedule	←→	307.45	Circadian Rhythm Sleep Disorder
F51.3	Sleepwalking (Somnambulism)	←→	307.46	Sleepwalking Disorder
F51.4	Sleep terrors (night terrors)	←→	307.46	Sleep Terror Disorder
F51.5	Nightmares	←→	307.47	Nightmare Disorder
F51.8	Other nonorganic sleep disorders	←		*No directly corresponding category, code as 307.47 Parasomnia NOS.*
F51.9	Nonorganic sleep disorder, unspecified		307.47	Dyssomnia NOS
F52	**Sexual Dysfunction, Not Caused By Organic Disorder or Disease**	Symptoms ≥ 6 months in the ICD-10.		**Sexual and Gender Identity Disorders**
F52.0	Lack or loss of sexual desire	←→	302.71	Hypoactive Sexual Desire Disorder
F52.1	Sexual aversion and lack of sexual enjoyment	←→		
F52.10	Sexual aversion	←→	302.79	Sexual Aversion Disorder
F52.11	Lack of sexual enjoyment	←		*No corresponding category, code as 302.70 Sexual Dysfunction NOS.*
F52.2	Failure of genital response	← → →	302.72 302.72	Male Erectile Disorder Female Sexual Arousal Disorder
F52.3	Orgasmic dysfunction	← → →	302.73 302.74	Female Orgasmic Disorder Male Orgasmic Disorder
F52.4	Premature ejaculation	←→	302.75	Premature Ejaculation
F52.5	Nonorganic vaginismus	←→	306.51	Vaginismus (Not Due to a General Medical Condition)

	ICD-10	cross-walk		DSM-IV-TR
F52	**Sexual Dysfunction, Not Caused By Organic Disorder or Disease**	Symptoms ≥ 6 months in the ICD-10.		**Sexual and Gender Identity Disorders**
F52.6	Nonorganic Dyspareunia	←——→	302.76	Dyspareunia (Not Due to a General Medical Condition)
F52.7	Excessive sexual drive	←——		*No corresponding category, code as 302.70 Sexual Dysfunction NOS.*
F52.8	Other sexual dysfunction, including: psychogenic dysmenorrhoe			
F52.9	Unspecified sexual dysfunction, not caused by organic disease or disorder	←——→	302.70	Sexual Dysfunction NOS
F53	**Mental and Behavioral Disorders Associated With the Puerperium, Not Elsewhere Classified**			
F53.0	Mild mental and behavioral disorders			*No corresponding category, code most likely as 300.9 Unspecified Mental Disorder (nonpsychotic). In particular cases refer also to 296.x Bipolar I Disorders ... With Postpartum Onset.*
F53.1	Severe mental and behavioral disorders			
F53.8	Other mental and behavioral disorders	←——		
F53.9	Puerperal mental disorder, unspecified			
F54	**Psychological and behavioral factors associated with disorders or diseases classified elsewhere**	←——→	316	**Psychological Factors Affecting a General Medical Condition**
F55	**Abuse of Non-Dependence-Producing Substances**			
F55.0	Antidepressants			
F55.1	Laxatives			
F55.2	Analgesics			
F55.3	Antacids	←——		*No corresponding category, code as 305.90 Other or Unknown Substance Abuse.*
F55.4	Vitamins			
F55.5	Steroids or hormones			
F55.6	Specific herbal or folk remedies			
F55.8	Other substances that do not produce dependence			
F55.9	Unspecified			
F59	**Unspecified Behavioral Syndromes Associated With Physiological Disturbances and Physical Factors**	←——		*No corresponding category, code as 316 Specified Psychological Factor Affecting ... [Indicate the General Medical Condition].*

	ICD-10	cross-walk		DSM-IV-TR
F6	**Disorders of Adult Personality and Behavior**			
F60	**Specific Personality Disorders**			**Personality Disorders**
F60.0	Paranoid personality disorder	←——→	301.00	Paranoid Personality Disorder
F60.1	Schizoid personality disorder	←——→	301.20	Schizoid Personality Disorder
F60.2	Dissocial personality disorder	←——→	301.7	Antisocial Personality Disorder
F60.3	Emotionally unstable personality disorder...			
F60.30	Impulsive type	←——		*No corresponding category, code as 301.9 Personality Disorder NOS.*
F60.31	Borderline type	←——→	301.83	Borderline Personality Disorder
F60.4	Histrionic personality disorder	←——→	301.50	Histrionic Personality Disorder
F60.5	Anankastic personality disorder	←——→	301.4	Obsessive-Compulsive Personality Disorder
F60.6	Anxious (avoidant) personality disorder	←——→	301.82	Avoidant Personality Disorder
F60.7	Dependent personality disorder	←——→	301.60	Dependent Personality Disorder
F60.8	Other specific personality disorders	←——		*No corresponding category, code as 301.9 Personality Disorder NOS.* *This includes also the Passive-Aggressive Personality Disorder – cf. Appendix B.*
F60.9	Personality disorder, unspecified	←——→	301.9	Personality Disorder NOS
F61	**Mixed and Other Personality Disorders**			
F61.0	Mixed personality disorders	←——		*No corresponding category, code as 301.9 Personality Disorder NOS.*
F61.1	Troublesome personality changes			
F62	**Enduring Personality Changes, Not Attributable to Brain Damage and Disease**			
F62.0	Enduring personality change after catastrophic experience			
F62.1	Enduring personality change after psychiatric illness	←——		*No corresponding category, code as 301.9 Personality Disorder NOS.*
F62.8	Other enduring personality changes			
F62.9	Enduring personality change, unspeci-fied			

	ICD-10		cross-walk		DSM-IV-TR
F63	**Habit and Impulse Disorders**		≥ 2 episodes within 12 months in the ICD-10, no comments in the DSM.		**Impulse-Control Disorders**
F63.0	Pathological gambling		←→	312.31	Pathological Gambling
F63.1	Pathological fire-setting (Pyromania)		←→	312.33	Pyromania
F63.2	Pathological stealing (Kleptomania)		←→	312.32	Kleptomania
F63.3	Trichotillomania		←→	312.39	Trichotillomania
F63.8	Other habit and impulse disorders		←		*No corresponding category, code as 312.30 Impulse-Control Disorder NOS.*
F63.9	Habit and impulse disorder, unspecified		←→	312.30	Impulse-Control Disorder NOS
F64	**Gender Identity Disorders**				**Gender Identity Disorders**
F64.0	Transsexualism		←→	302.85	Gender Identity Disorder in Adolescents or Adults
F64.1	Dual-role transvestism		←		*No corresponding category, code as 302.6 Gender Identity Disorder NOS.*
F64.2	Gender identity disorder of childhood		←→	302.6	Gender Identity Disorder in Children
F64.8	Other gender identity disorders		←		*No corresponding category, code as 302.6 Gender Identity Disorder NOS.*
F64.9	Gender identity disorder, unspecified		←→	302.6	Gender Identity Disorder NOS
F65	**Disorders of Sexual Preference**				**Paraphilias**
F65.0	Fetishisms		←→	302.81	Fetishism
F65.1	Fetishistic transvestism		←→	302.3	Transvestic Fetishism
F65.2	Exhibitionism		←→	302.4	Exhibitionism
F65.3	Voyeurism		←→	302.82	Voyeurism
F65.4	Paedophilia		←→	302.2	Pedophilia
F65.5	Sadomasochism		← → →	302.83 302.84	Sexual Masochism Sexual Sadism
F65.6	Multiple disorders of sexual preference		←		*No corresponding category, code as 302.9 Paraphila NOS.*
F65.8	Other disorders of sexual preference				
F65.9	Disorder of sexual preference, unspecified		←	302.9	Paraphilia NOS

	ICD-10	cross-walk		DSM-IV-TR
F66	**Psychological and Behavioral Disorders Associated With Sexual Development and Orientation**			
	F66.x0 Heterosexuality F66.x1 Homosexuality F66.x2 Bisexuality F66.x8 Other, including prepubertal	← In ICD-10, the 5th character marks sexual orientation.		*No corresponding category.*
F66.0	Sexual maturation disorder			
F66.1	Egodystonic sexual orientation			
F66.2	Sexual relationship disorder	←		*No corresponding category, code as 302.9 Sexual Disorder NOS.*
F66.8	Other psychosexual development disorders			
F66.9	Psychosexual development disorder			
F68	**Other Disorders of Adult Personality and Behavior**			
F68.0	Elaboration of physical symptoms for psychological reasons	←		*No corresponding category, code as 300.9 Unspecified Mental Disorder (nonpsychotic), possibly also consider 300.82 Undifferentiated Somatoform Disorder.*
F68.1	Intentional production or feigning of symptoms or disabilities, either physical or psychological (factitious disorder)	←→	300.19	Factitious Disorder ... NOS
F68.8	Other specified disorders of adult personality and behavior	←		*No corresponding category, code as 300.9 Unspecified Mental Disorder (nonpsychotic).*
F69	**Unspecified Disorder of Adult Personality and Behavior**	←		*No corresponding category, code as 300.9 Unspecified Mental Disorder (nonpsychotic).*
F7	**Mental Retardation**			**Mental Retardation**
	F7x.0 No, or minimal, impairment of behavior F7x.1 Significant impairment of behavior requiring attention or treatment F7x.8 Other impairments of behavior F7x.9 Without mention of impairment of behavior	The 4th character of the ICD-10 classifies the extent of the mental retardation.		*No corresponding category.*

	ICD-10	cross-walk		DSM-IV-TR
F7	**Mental Retardation**	**Continuation**		**Mental Retardation**
F70	Mild mental retardation	←→	317	Mild Mental Retardation
F71	Moderate mental retardation	←→	318.0	Moderate Mental Retardation
F72	Severe mental retardation	←→	318.1	Severe Mental Retardation
F73	Profound mental retardation	←→	318.2	Profound Mental Retardation
F78	Other mental retardation	←		*No corresponding category, code as 319 Mental Retardation …*
F79	Unspecified mental retardation	←→	319	Mental Retardation, Severity Unspecified
F8	**Disorder of Psychological Development**			**Disorder Usually First Diagnosed in Infancy, Childhood, or Adolescence**
F80	**Specific Developmental Disorders of Speech and Language**			**Communication Disorders**
F80.0	Specific speech articulation disorder	←→	315.39	Phonological Disorder
F80.1	Expressive language disorder	←→	315.31	Expressive Language Disorder
F80.2	Receptive language disorder	←→	315.31	Mixed Receptive-Expressive Language Disorder
F80.3	Acquired aphasia with epilepsy (Landau-Kleffner syndrome)	←		*No corresponding category, code as 307.9 Communication Disorder NOS.*
F80.8	Other developmental disorders of speech and language			
F80.9	Developmental disorder of speech and language, unspecified	←→	307.9	Communication Disorder NOS
F81	**Specific Developmental Disorders of Scholastic Skills**			**Learning Disorders**
F81.0	Specific reading disorder	←→	315.00	Reading Disorder
F81.1	Specific spelling disorder	←		*No corresponding category, code as 315.9 Learning Disorder NOS.*
F81.2	Specific disorder of arithmetical skills	←→	315.1	Mathematics Disorder
F81.3	Mixed disorder of scholastic skills	←		*No corresponding category, code as 315.9 Learning Disorder NOS.*
F81.8	Other Developmental Disorders of scholastic skills			
F81.9	Developmental disorder of scholastic skills, unspecified	←→	315.9	Learning Disorder NOS
F82	**Specific Developmental Disorder of Motor Function**	←→	315.4	**Developmental Coordination Disorder**

	ICD-10	cross-walk		DSM-IV-TR
F83	Mixed Specific Developmental Disorders	←		*No corresponding category, code as 313.9 Disorder of Infancy, Childhood, or Adolescence NOS.*
F84	Pervasive Developmental Disorders			**Pervasive Developmental Disorders**
F84.0	Childhood autism	←→	299.00	Autistic Disorder
F84.1	Atypical autism	←		*No corresponding category, code as 299.80 Pervasive Developmental Disorder NOS.*
F84.2	Rett's syndrome	←→	299.80	Rett's Disorder
F84.3	Other childhood disintegrative disorder	←→	299.10	Childhood Disintegrative Disorder
F84.4	Overactive disorder associated with mental retardation and stereotyped movements	←		*No corresponding category, code as 313.9 Disorder of Infancy, Childhood, or Adolescence NOS*
F84.5	Asperger's syndrome	←→	299.80	Asperger's Disorder
F84.8	Other pervasive developmental disorders	←		*No corresponding category, code as 313.9 Disorder of Infancy, Childhood, or Adolescence NOS*
F84.9	Pervasive developmental disorders, unspecified	←→	299.80	Pervasive Developmental Disorder NOS
F88	Other Disorders of Psychological Development	←		
F89	Unspecified Disorder of Psychological Development			
F9	Behavioral and Emotional Disorders With Onset Usually Occurring in Childhood and Adolescence			**Attention-Deficit and Disruptive Behavior Disorders**
F90	Hyperkinetic Disorders			**Attention-Deficit/Hyperactivity Disorder**
F90.0	Disturbance of activity and attention	←		*No directly corresponding category, if not definitely attributable to 314.0x code as 314.9 Attention-Deficit/Hyperactivity Disorder NOS.*
F90.1	Hyperkinetic conduct disorder	←		*No directly corresponding category, possibly code as 314.0x Attention-Deficit/Hyperactivity Disorder and 312.8 Conduct Disorder.* *Otherwise code as 314.9 Attention-Deficit/Hyperactivity Disorder NOS.*
F90.8	Other hyperkinetic disorders	←		*No corresponding category, code as 314.9 Attention-Deficit/Hyperactivity Disorder NOS.*
F90.9	Hyperkinetic disorder, unspecified	←→	314.9	Attention-Deficit/Hyperactivity Disorder NOS

	ICD-10		cross-walk		DSM-IV-TR	
F91	**Conduct Disorders**		←——→	**312.8**	**Conduct Disorder**	
F91.0	Conduct disorder confined to the family context					
F91.1	Unsocialized conduct disorder		←——		*No corresponding differentiation.*	
F91.2	Socialized conduct disorder					
F91.3	Oppositional defiant disorder		←——→	313.81	Oppositional Defiant Disorder	
F91.8	Other conduct disorders		←——		*No corresponding category, code as 312.9 Disruptive Behavior Disorder NOS.*	
F91.9	Conduct disorder, unspecified		←——→	312.9	Disruptive Behavior Disorder NOS	
F92	**Mixed Disorders of Conduct and Emotions**					
F92.0	Depressive conduct disorder				*No corresponding category, maybe code as. 312.8 Conduct Disorder and additional disorder, otherwise 300.9 Unspecified Mental Disorder (nonpsychotic).*	
F92.8	Other mixed disorders of conduct and emotions		←——			
F92.9	Mixed disorder of conduct and emotions, unspecified					
F93	**Emotional Disorders With Onset Specific to Childhood**					
F93.0	Separation anxiety disorder of childhood		←——→	309.21	Separation Anxiety Disorder	
F93.1	Phobic anxiety disorder of childhood		←——		*No directly corresponding category, for F93.1 possibly also code 300.22 or 300.29, for F93.2 maybe also 300.23 (cf. Anxiety Disorders), otherwise code as 313.9 Disorder of Infancy, Childhood, or Adolescence NOS.*	
F93.2	Social anxiety disorder of childhood					
F93.3	Sibling rivalry disorder		←——→	V61.8	Sibling Relational Problem	
F93.8	Other childhood emotional disorders		←——		*No corresponding category, code as 313.9 Disorder of Infancy, Childhood, or Adolescence NOS.*	
F93.9	Childhood emotional disorder, unspecified					
F94	**Disorder of Social Functioning With Onset Specific to Childhood and Adolescence**					
F94.0	Elective mutism		←——→		Selective Mutism	
F94.1	Reactive attachment disorder of childhood		←——→		Reactive Attachment Disorder of Infancy or Early Childhood Inhibited Type	
F94.2	Disinhibited attachment disorder of childhood		←——→		Disinhibited Type	

	ICD-10	cross-walk		DSM-IV-TR
F94	**Disorder of Social Functioning With Onset Specific to Childhood and Adolescence**	**continuation**		
F94.8	Other childhood disorders of social functioning	←		*No corresponding category, code as 313.9 Disorder of Infancy, Childhood, or Adolescence NOS.*
F94.9	Childhood disorder of social functioning, unspecified			
F95	**Tic Disorders**			**Tic Disorders**
F95.0	Transient tic disorder	←→	307.21	Transient Tic Disorder
F95.1	Chronic motor or vocal tic disorder	←→	307.22	Chronic Motor or Vocal Tic Disorder
F95.2	Combined vocal and multiple motor tic disorder (de la Tourette's disorder)	←→	307.23	Tourette's Disorder
F95.8	Other tic disorders	←		*No corresponding category, code as 307.21 Tic Disorder NOS.*
F95.9	Tic disorder, unspecified	←→	307.21	Tic Disorder NOS
F98	**Other behavioral and Emotional Disorders With Onset Usually Occurring in Childhood and Adolescence**			
F98.0	Nonorganic enuresis	←→	307.6	Enuresis
F98.1	Nonorganic encopresis	←→	307.7	Encopresis Without Constipation and Overflow Incontinence
F98.2	Feeding disorder of infancy and childhood (including Rumination disorder)	←——→	307.59 307.53	Feeding Disorder of Infancy or Early Childhood Rumination Disorder
F98.3	Pica of infancy and childhood	←→	307.52	Pica
F98.4	Stereotyped movement disorder	←→	307.3	Stereotypic Movement Disorder
F98.5	Stuttering (stammering)	←→	307.0	Stuttering
F98.6	Cluttering	←		*No corresponding category, code most likely as 307.9 Communication Disorder NOS.*
F98.8	Other specified behavioral and emotional disorder with onset usually occurring in childhood and adolescence	←		*No corresponding category, code as 313.9 Disorder of Infancy Childhood, or Adolescence NOS ...*
F98.9	Unspecified behavioral and emotional disorder with onset usually occurring in childhood and adolescence	←→	313.9	Disorder of Infancy, Childhood, or Adolescence NOS
F99	**Unspecified Mental Disorder**	←→	**300.9**	**Unspecified Mental Disorder (nonpsychotic)**

DSM-IV-TR – ICD-10

	DSM-IV-TR	cross-walk		ICD-10
	Disorders Usually First Diagnosed in Infancy, Childhood, or Adolescence			
	Mental Retardation		**F7**	**Mental Retardation**
317	Mild Mental Retardation	←——→	F70.9	Mild mental retardation with unspecified impairment of behavior
318.0	Moderate Mental Retardation	←——→	F71.9	Moderate mental retardation with unspecified impairment of behavior
318.1	Severe Mental Retardation	←——→	F72.9	Severe mental retardation with unspecified impairment of behavior
318.2	Profound Mental Retardation	←——→	F73.9	Profound mental retardation with unspecified impairment of behavior
319	Mental Retardation, Severity Unspecified	←——→	F79.9	Unspecified mental retardation
	Learning Disorders		**F8**	**Disorders of Psychological Development**
			F81	**Specific Developmental Disorders of Scholastic Skills**
315.00	Reading Disorder	←——→	F81.0	Specific reading disorder
315.1	Mathematics Disorder	←——→	F81.2	Specific disorder of arithmetical skills
315.2	Disorder of Written Expression	←——	No corresponding category, code as *F81.8 Other developmental disorder of scholastic skills.*	
315.9	Learning Disorder OS	←——→	F81.9	Developmental disorder of scholastic skills, unspecified
	Motor Skills Disorder			
315.4	Developmental Coordination Disorder	←——→	F82	Specific developmental disorder of motor function
	Communication Disorders		**F80**	**Specific Developmental Disorders of Speech and Language**
315.31	Expressive Language Disorder	←——→	F80.1	Expressive language disorder
315.31	Mixed Receptive-Expressive Disorder	←——→	F80.2	Receptive language disorder
315.39	Phonological Disorder	←——→	F80.0	Specific speech articulation disorder
307.0	Stuttering	←——→	F98.5	Other behavioral and emotional disorders with onset usually occurring in childhood and adolescence: Stuttering (stammering)

	DSM-IV-TR	cross-walk		ICD-10
	Communication Disorders	continuation	**F80**	**Specific Developmental Disorders of Speech and Language**
307.9	Communication Disorder OS	←——→	F80.9	Developmental disorder of speech and language, unspecified
	Pervasive Developmental Disorders	←——→	**F84**	**Pervasive Developmental Disorders**
299.00	Autistic Disorder	←——→	F84.0	Childhood autism
299.80	Rett's Disorder	←——→	F84.2	Rett's syndrome
299.10	Childhood Disintegrative Disorder	←——→	F84.3	Other childhood disintegrative disorder
299.80	Asperger's Disorder	←——→	F84.5	Asperger's syndrome
299.80	Pervasive Developmental Disorder NOS		F84.9	Pervasive developmental disorder, unspecified
	Attention-Deficit and Disruptive Behavior Disorders		**F9**	**Behavioral and Emotional Disorders With Onset Usually Occurring in Childhood and Adolescence**
314.xx	Attention-Deficit/Hyperactivity Disorder		F90	Hyperkinetic disorders
314.01	Combined Type			*No directly corresponding category, if not able to definitely relate to ...*
314.00	Predominantly Inattentive Type	←——		*F90.0 Disturbance of activity and attention or F98.8 Other emotional and behavioral disorders ... Attention disorder without hyperactivity or*
314.01	Predominantly Hyperactive-Impulsive Type			*F90.1 Hyperkinetic conduct disorder code as F90.9 Hyperkinetic disorder, unspecified.*
314.9	Attention-Deficit/Hyperactivity Disorder	←——→	F90.9	Hyperkinetic disorder, unspecified
312.8	Conduct Disorder	←——		*No directly corresponding category, if not able to definitely relate to ...*
312.81	Childhood-Onset Type			*F91.0 Conduct disorder confined to the family context or*
312.82	Adolescent-Onset Type			*F91.1 Unsocialized conduct disorder or*
312.89	Unspecified Onset Type			*F91.2 Socialized conduct disorder code as F91.9 Conduct disorder, unspecified.*
	... mild ... moderate ... severe	←—— Additional differentiation in the DSM without separate codes.		*No corresponding differentiation.*

	DSM-IV-TR	cross-walk		ICD-10
	Attention-Deficit and Disruptive Behavior Disorders	continuation	**F9**	**Behavioral and Emotional Disorders With Onset Usually Occurring in Childhood and Adolescence**
313.81	Oppositional Defiant Disorder	←——→	F91.3	Oppositional defiant disorder
312.9	Disruptive Behavior Disorder NOS	←——→	F91.9	Conduct disorder, unspecified
	Feeding and Eating Disorders of Infancy or Early Childhood		**In: F98**	**Other Emotional and Behavioral Disorders With Onset Usually Occurring in Childhood and Adolescence**
307.52	Pica	←——→	F98.3	Pica of infancy and childhood
307.53	Rumination Disorder	←——		*No directly corresponding category, code as F98.2 Feeding disorder of infancy and childhood.*
307.59	Feeding Disorder of Infancy or Early Childhood		F98.2	Feeding disorder of infancy and childhood
	Tic Disorders		**F95**	**Tic Disorders**
307.23	Tourette's Disorder	←——→	F95.2	Combined vocal and multiple motor tic disorder (de la Tourette's syndrome)
307.22	Chronic Motor or Vocal Tic Disorder	←——→	F95.1	Chronic motor or vocal tic disorder
307.21	Transient Tic Disorder Single Episode Recurrent	←—— *Additional differentiation in the DSM without separate codes.*	F95.0	Transient tic disorder *No corresponding differentiation.*
307.20	Tic Disorder NOS	←——→	F95.9	Tic disorder, unspecified
	Elimination Disorders		**In: F98**	**Other Behavioral and Emotional Disorders With Onset Usually Occurring in Childhood and Adolescence**
787.6	Encopresis With Constipation and Overflow Incontinence	←——		*No directly corresponding category, code as R15 faecal incontinence.*
307.7	Without Constipation and Overflow Incontinence	←——→	F98.1	Nonorganic encopresis
307.6	Enuresis (Not Due to a General Medical Condition) Nocturnal Only Diurnal Only Nocturnal and Diurnal	←—— *Additional differentiation in the DSM without separate codes.*	F98.0	Nonorganic enuresis *No corresponding differentiation.*

	DSM-IV-TR	cross-walk		ICD-10
	Disorders Usually First Diagnosed in Infancy, Childhood, or Adolescence			
309.21	Separation Anxiety Disorder	←——→	F93.0	Separation anxiety disorder of childhood
	Early Onset	←—— *Additional differentiation in the DSM without separate codes.*		*No corresponding differentiation.*
313.23	Selective Mutism	←——→	F94.0	Elective mutism
313.89	Reactive Attachment Disorder of Infancy or Early Childhood			
	Inhibited Type	←——→	F94.1	Reactive attachment disorder of childhood
	Disinhibited Type	←——→	F94.2	Disinhibited attachment disorder of childhood
307.3	Stereotypic Movement Disorder With Self-Injurious Behavior	←——→	F98.4	Stereotyped movement disorder
		←—— *Additional differentiation in the DSM without separate codes.*		*No corresponding differentiation.*
313.9	Disorder of Infancy, Childhood, or Adolescence NOS	←——→	F98.9	*Unspecified behavioral and emotional disorders with onset usually occurring in childhood and adolescence.*
	Delirium, Dementia, and Amnestic and Other Cognitive Disorders			**Organic, Including Symptomatic, Mental Disorders**
	Delirium		F05	**Delirium, Not Induced By Alcohol and Other Psychoactive Substances**
293.0	Delirium Due to ... *[Indicate the General Medical Condition]*	←—— ←——		*No directly corresponding category. Whenever it is known that a dementia exists code as* F05.0 *Delirium, not superimposed on dementia* or F05.1 *Delirium, superimposed on dementia, otherwise code as* F05.9 *Delirium, unspecified.*
--.-	*Substance-Induced Delirium (for substance-specific codes refer to Substance-Related Disorders)*		--.-	
-- -	*Substance Withdrawal Delirium (for substance-specific codes refer to Substance-Related Disorders)*		--.-	
780.09	**Delirium NOS**		F05.9	Delirium, unspecified

	DSM-IV-TR	cross-walk		ICD-10
294.1x	**Dementia of the Alzheimer's Type**		**F00.x**	**Dementia in Alzheimer's Disease**
294.1	... Without Behavioral Disturbance	←		*No corresponding differentiation.*
294.11	... With Behavioral Disturbance			
	With Early Onset	←→	F00.0	Dementia in Alzheimer's disease with early onset
	With Late Onset	←→	F00.1	Dementia in Alzheimer's disease with late onset
290.4x	**Vascular Dementia**		**F01**	**Vascular Dementia**
	... With Behavioral Disturbance	←		
		Additional differentiation in the DSM without separate codes.		*No corresponding differentiation.*
290.40	Uncomplicated	←		*No directly corresponding category, code as F01.08 Other vascular dementia ... without additional symptoms.*
290.41	With Delirium	←		*No directly corresponding category, code as F01.0 Vascular dementia of acute onset and F05.1 delirium, superimposed on dementia.*
290.42	With Delusions	←		*No directly corresponding category, code as F01.01 Other vascular dementia ... with other symptoms, predominantly delusional.*
290.43	With Depressed Mood	←		*No directly corresponding category, code as F01.03 Other vascular dementia ... with other symptoms, predominantly depressive.*
294.1x	**Dementia Due to ....** [Indicate the General Medical Condition]	←→		*If no corresponding category (see below) can be found, code as F02.8 Dementia in Other Specified Diseases Classified Elsewhere.*
294.10	... Without Behavioral Disturbance			
294.11	... With Behavioral Disturbance	←		*No corresponding differentiation.*
	Dementia Due to HIV Disease	←→	F02.4	Dementia in Human Immunodeficiency Virus (HIV) disease
	Dementia Due to Head Trauma	←		*No corresponding category, code as F02.8 Dementia in Other Specified Diseases Classified Elsewhere.*
	Dementia Due to Parkinson's Disease	←→	F02.3	Dementia in Parkinson's disease
	Dementia Due to Huntington's Disease	←→	F02.2	Dementia in Huntington's disease
	Dementia Due to Pick's Disease	←→	F02.0	Dementia in Pick's disease
	Dementia Due to Creutzfeld-Jakob Disease	←→	F02.1	Dementia in Creutzfeld-Jakob disease
— -	*Substance-Induced Persisting Dementia (for substance-specific codes refer to Substance-Related Disorders)*		—.-	
294.8	Dementia NOS	←→	F03	Unspecified dementia

	DSM-IV-TR	cross-walk		ICD-10
	Amnestic Disorders			
294.0	Amnestic Disorder Due to ... [Indicate the General Medical Condition]	←——→	F04	Organic amnesic syndrome, not induced by alcohol and other psychoactive substances
	Transient Chronic	←—— Additional differentiation in the DSM without separate codes.		No corresponding differentiation.
--.-	Substance-Induced Persisting Amnestic Disorder (for substance-specific codes refer to Substance-Related Disorders)		—.-	
294.8	Amnestic Disorder NOS	←——		No directly corresponding category, most likely code as R41.3, not F04.
	Other Cognitive Disorders			
294.9	Cognitive Disorder NOS	←——		No directly corresponding category, most likely code as F06.9 Unspecified mental disorder due to brain damage and dysfunction and to physical disease consider F06.7 Mild cognitive disorder F06.70 Not associated with a physical disorder F06.71 Associated with a physical disorder F07.1 Postencephalitic syndrome F07.2 Postconcussional syndrome F07.8 Other organic personality and behavioral disorders ...
	Mental Disorders Due to a General Medical Condition			
293.89	Catatonic Disorder Due to... [Indicate the General Medical Condition]	←——→	F06.1	Organic catatonic disorder
310.1	Personality Change Due to... [Indicate the General Medical Condition] Labile Type Disinhibited Type Aggressive Type Apathetic Type Paranoid Type Other Type Combined Type Unspecified Type	←——→ ←—— Additional differentiation in the DSM without separate codes.	F07.0	Organic personality disorder No corresponding differentiation.
293.9	Mental Disorder NOS Due to... [Indicate the General Medical Condition]		F09	Unspecified organic or symptomatic mental disorder

	DSM-IV-TR	cross-walk		ICD-10
	Substance-Related Disorders		**F1**	**Mental and Behavioral Disorders Due to Psychoactive Substance Use**
	Alcohol-Related Disorders		**F10**	**Disorders Due to Use of Alcohol**
	Alcohol Use Disorders			
303.90	Alcohol Dependence	←——→	F10.2	Dependence syndrome
	With Physiological Dependence Without Physiological Dependence Early Full Remission Early Partial Remission Sustained Full Remission Sustained Partial Remission	←—— Additional differentiation in the DSM without separate codes.		*No corresponding differentiation.*
	On Agonist Therapy	←——→	F10.22	Currently on a clinically supervised maintenance or replacement regime
	In a Controlled Environment	←——→	F10.21	Currently abstinent but in a protected environment
305.00	Alcohol Abuse	←——→	F10.1	Harmful use
	Alcohol-Induced Disorders			
303.00	Alcohol Intoxication	←——→	F10.0	Acute intoxication
291.81	Alcohol Withdrawal	←——→	F10.3	Withdrawal state
	... With Perceptual Disturbances	←—— Additional differentiation in the DSM without separate codes.		*No corresponding differentiation.*
291.0	Alcohol Intoxication Delirium	←——→	F10.03	Acute intoxication ... With delirium
291.0	Alcohol Withdrawal Delirium	←——→	F10.4	Withdrawal state with delirium
291.2	Alcohol-Induced Persisting Dementia	←——→	F10.73	Residual and late-onset psychotic disorder ... Dementia
291.1	Alcohol-Induced Persisting Amnestic Disorder	←——→	F10.6	Amnesic syndrome
291.5 291.3	Alcohol-Induced Psychotic Disorders ... With Delusions ... With Hallucinations	←——→	F10.51 F10.52	Psychotic disorder ... Predominantly delusional Psychotic disorder... Predominantly hallucinatory
	... With Onset During Intoxication ... With Onset During Withdrawal	←—— Additional differentiation in the DSM without separate codes.		*No corresponding differentiation.*

	DSM-IV-TR	cross-walk		ICD-10
	Alcohol-Related Disorders	**Continuation**	**F10**	**Disorders Due to Use of Alcohol**
291.89	Alcohol-Induced Mood Disorder	←		*No corresponding category, code as F10.8 Other mental and behavioral disorders, except for ...*
	... With Depressive Features	←→	F10.54	Psychotic disorder... Predominantly depressive symptoms
	... With Manic Features	←→	F10.55	Psychotic disorder... Predominantly manic symptoms
	... With Mixed Features	←→	F10.56	Psychotic disorder... Mixed
	... With Onset During Intoxication ... With Onset During Withdrawal	← Additional differentiation in the DSM without separate codes.		*No corresponding differentiation.*
291.89	Alcohol-Induced Anxiety Disorder ... With Generalized Anxiety ... With Panic Attacks ... With Obsessive-Compulsive Symptoms ... With Phobic Symptoms ... With Onset During Intoxication ... With Onset During Withdrawal	← Additional differentiation in the DSM without separate codes.		*No corresponding category, code as F10.8 Other mental and behavioral disorders.*
291.89	Alcohol-Induced Sexual Dysfunction ... With Impaired Desire ... With Impaired Arousal ... With Impaired Orgasm ... With Sexual Pain ... With Onset During Intoxication	← Additional differentiation in the DSM without separate codes.		*No corresponding category, code as F10.8 Other mental and behavioral disorders.*
291.89	Alcohol-Induced Sleep Disorder ... Insomnia Type ... Hypersomnia Type ... Parasomnia Type ... Mixed Type ... With Onset During Intoxication ... With Onset During Withdrawal	← Additional differentiation in the DSM without separate codes.		*No corresponding category, code as F10.8 Other mental and behavioral disorders.*
291.9	Alcohol-Related Disorder NOS	←→	F10.9	Unspecified mental and behavioral disorder

	DSM-IV-TR	cross-walk		ICD-10
	Amphetamine (or Amphetamine-Like)-Related Disorders		**F15**	**Disorders Due to Use of Other Stimulants, Including Caffeine**
	Amphetamine Use Disorders			
304.40	Amphetamine Dependence	←——→	F15.2	Dependence syndrome
	With Physiological Dependence Without Physiological Dependence Early Full Remission Early Partial Remission Sustained Full Remission Sustained Partial Remission On Agonist Therapy	←—— Additional differentiation in the DSM without separate codes. ←——→		*No corresponding differentiation.*
			F15.22	Currently on a clinically supervised maintenance or replacement regime
			F15.21	Currently abstinent but in a protected environment
	In a Controlled Environment	←——→	F15.1	Harmful use
305.70	Amphetamine Abuse	←——→		
	Amphetamine-Induced Disorders			
292.89	Amphetamine Intoxication	←——→	F15.0	Acute intoxication
	... With Perceptual Disturbances	←——→ Additional differentiation in the DSM without separate codes.	F15.04	... With perceptional distortions
292.0	Amphetamine Withdrawal	←——→	F15.3	Withdrawal state
292.81	Amphetamine Intoxication Delirium	←——→	F15.03	Acute intoxication... With delirium
292.11	Amphetamine-Induced Psychotic Disorder With Delusions	←——→		
			F15.51	Psychotic disorder ... Predominantly delusional
292.12	With Hallucinations	←——→	F15.52	Psychotic disorder ... Predominantly hallucinatory
	... With Onset During Intoxication	←—— Additional differentiation in the DSM without separate codes.		
292.84	Amphetamine-Induced Mood Disorder	←——		*No corresponding category, code as F15.8 Other mental and behavioral disorders, except for*
	... With Depressive Features	←——→	F15.54	Psychotic disorder ... Pred. depressive symptoms
	... With Manic Features	←——→	F15.55	Psychotic disorder ... Pred. manic symptoms
	... With Mixed Features	←——→	F15.56	Psychotic disorder ... Mixed
	... With Onset During Intoxication ... With Onset During Withdrawal	←—— Additional differentiation in the DSM without separate codes.		*No corresponding differentiation.*

	DSM-IV-TR	cross-walk		ICD-10
	Amphetamine-Related Disorders	**Continuation**	**F15**	**Disorders Due to Use of Other Stimulants, Including Caffeine**
292.89	Amphetamine-Induced Anxiety Disorder ... With Generalized Anxiety ... With Panic Attacks ... With Obsessive-Compulsive Symptoms ... With Phobic Symptoms ... With Onset During Intoxication	← Additional differentiation in the DSM without separate codes.		*No corresponding category, code as F15.8 Other mental and behavioral disorders.*
292.89	Amphetamine-Induced Sexual Dysfunction ... With Impaired Desire ... With Impaired Arousal ... With Impaired Orgasm ... With Sexual Pain ... With Onset During Intoxication	← Additional differentiation in the DSM without separate codes.		*No corresponding category, code as F15.8 Other mental and behavioral disorders.*
292.89	Amphetamine-Induced Sleep Disorder ... Insomnia Type ... Hypersomnia Type ... Parasomnia Type ... Mixed Type ... With Onset During Intoxication ... With Onset During Withdrawal	← Additional differentiation in the DSM without separate codes.		*No corresponding category, code as F15.8 Other mental and behavioral disorders.*
292.9	Amphetamine-Related Disorder NOS	←→	F15.9	Unspecified mental and behavioral disorders
	Cannabis-Related Disorders		**F12**	**Disorders Due to Use of Cannabinoids**
	Cannabis Use Disorders			
304.30	Cannabis Dependence	←→	F12.2	Dependence syndrome
	With Physiological Dependence Without Physiological Dependence Early Full Remission Early Partial Remission Sustained Full Remission Sustained Partial Remission In a Controlled Environment	← Additional differentiation in the DSM without separate codes. ←→	 F12.21	*No corresponding differentiation.* Currently abstinent but in a protected environment
305.20	Cannabis Abuse	←→	F12.1	Harmful use

	DSM-IV-TR	cross-walk		ICD-10
	Cannabis-Related Disorders	Continuation	F10	Disorders Due to Use of Cannabinoids
	Cannabis-Induced Disorders			
292.89	Cannabis Intoxication	←——→	F12.0	Acute intoxication
	... With Perceptual Disturbances	←——→	F12.04	... With perceptional distortions
		Additional differentiation in the DSM without separate codes.		
292.81	Cannabis Intoxication Delirium	←——→	F12.03	Acute intoxication... With delirium
291.5 291.3	Cannabis-Induced Psychotic Disorder ... With Delusions ... With Hallucinations	←——→ ←——→	F12.51 F12.52	Psychotic Disorder ... Predominantly delusional Psychotic Disorder ... Predominantly hallucinatory
	... With Onset During Intoxication	←——		
		Additional differentiation in the DSM without separate codes.		
291.8	Cannabis-Induced Anxiety Disorder ... With Generalized Anxiety ... With Panic Attacks ... With Obsessive-Compulsive Symptoms ... With Phobic Symptoms ... With Onset During Intoxication	←—— Additional differentiation in the DSM without separate codes. ←——→	*No corresponding category, code as F12.8 Other mental and behavioral disorders.*	
291.9	Cannabis-Related Disorder NOS		F12.9	Unspecified mental and behavioral disorders
	Hallucinogen-Related Disorders		F16	**Disorders Due to Use of Hallucinogens**
	Hallucinogen Use Disorder			
304.50	Hallucinogen Dependence	←——→	F16.2	Dependence syndrome
	Early Full Remission Early Partial Remission Sustained Full Remission Sustained Partial Remission	←—— Additional differentiation in the DSM without separate codes.	*No corresponding differentiation.*	
	In a Controlled Environment	←——→	F16.21	Currently abstinent but in a protected environment
305.30	Hallucinogen Abuse	←——→	F16.1	Harmful use
	Hallucinogen-Induced Disorders			
292.89	Hallucinogen Intoxication	←——→	F16.0	Acute intoxication
292.89	Hallucinogen Persisting Perception Disorder (flashback)	←——→	F16.70	Residual and late-onset psychotic disorder ... Flashbacks

DSM-IV-TR		cross-walk		ICD-10	
Hallucinogen-Related Disorders		**Continuation**	**F16**	**Disorders Due to Use of Hallucinogens**	
292.81	Hallucinogen Intoxication Delirium	←——→	F16.03	Acute intoxication ... With delirium	
	Hallucinogen-Induced Psychotic Disorders				
292.11	... With Delusions	←——→	F16.51	Psychotic Disorder ... Predominantly delusional	
292.12	... With Hallucinations	←——→	F16.52	Psychotic Disorder... Predominantly hallucinatory	
	... With Onset During Intoxication	←—— Additional differentiation in the DSM without separate codes.			
292.84	Hallucinogen-Induced Mood Disorder	←——		*No corresponding category, code as F16.8 Other mental and behavioral disorders, except for*	
	... With Depressive Features	←——→	F16.54	Psychotic Disorder... Predominantly depressive symptoms	
	... With Manic Features	←——→	F16.55	Psychotic Disorder... Predominantly manic symptoms	
	... With Mixed Features	←——→	F16.56	Psychotic Disorder... Mixed	
	... With Onset During Intoxication	←—— Additional differentiation in the DSM without separate codes.		*No corresponding differentiation.*	
292.89	Hallucinogen-Induced Anxiety Disorder ... With Generalized Anxiety ... With Panic Attacks ... With Obsessive-Compulsive Symptoms ... With Phobic Symptoms ... With Onset During Intoxication ... With Onset During Withdrawal	←—— Additional differentiation in the DSM without separate codes.		*No corresponding category, code as F16.8 Other mental and behavioral disorders.*	
292.9	Hallucinogen-Related Disorder NOS	←——→	F16.9	Unspecified mental and behavioral disorder	
Inhalant-Related Disorders			**F18**	**Disorders Due to Use of Volatile Solvents**	
Inhalant Use Disorder					
304.60	Inhalant Dependence	←——→	F18.2	Dependence syndrome	
	Early Full Remission Early Partial Remission Sustained Full Remission Sustained Partial Remission	←—— Additional differentiation in the DSM without separate codes.		*No corresponding differentiation.*	
	In a Controlled Environment	←——→	F18.21	Currently abstinent but in a protected environment	
305.90	Inhalant Abuse	←——→	F18.1	Harmful use	

43

	DSM-IV-TR	cross-walk		ICD-10
	Inhalant-Related Disorders	**Continuation**	**F18**	**Disorders Due to Use of Volatile Solvents**
	Inhalant-Induced Disorders			
292.89	Inhalant Intoxication	←→	F18.0	Acute intoxication
292.81	Inhalant Intoxication Delirium	←→	F18.03	Acute intoxication ... With delirium
292.82	Inhalant-Induced Persisting Dementia	←→	F18.73	Residual and late-onset psychotic disorder ... Dementia
292.11 292.12	Inhalant-Induced Psychotic Disorder ... With Delusions ... With Hallucinations ... With Onset During Intoxication	←→ ←→ ← Additional differentiation in the DSM without separate codes.	F18.51 F18.52	Psychotic disorder ... Predominantly delusional Psychotic disorder... Predominantly hallucinatory
292.84	Inhalant-Induced Mood Disorder	←		*No corresponding category, code as F15.8 Other mental and behavioral disorders, except for*
	... With Depressive Features ... With Manic Features ... With Mixed Features ... With Onset During Intoxication	←→ ←→ ←→ ← Additional differentiation in the DSM without separate codes.	F18.54 F18.55 F18.56	Psychotic disorder ... Predominantly depressive symptoms Psychotic disorder... Predominantly manic sympt. Psychotic disorder... Mixed *No corresponding differentiation.*
292.89	Inhalant-Induced Anxiety Disorder ... With Generalized Anxiety ... With Panic Attacks ... With Obsessive-Compulsive Symptoms ... With Phobic Symptoms ... With Onset During Intoxication	← Additional differentiation in the DSM without separate codes.		*No corresponding category, code as F18.8 Other mental and behavioral disorders.*
292.9	Inhalant-Related Disorder NOS	←→	F18.9	Unspecified mental and behavioral disorder
	Caffeine-Related Disorders		**F15**	**Disorders Due to Use of Other Stimulants, Including Caffeine**
	Caffeine-Induced Disorders			
305.90	Caffeine Intoxication	←→	F15.0	Acute intoxication
292.89	Caffeine-Induced Anxiety Disorder ... With Generalized Anxiety ... With Panic Attacks ... With Obsessive-Compulsive Symptoms ... With Phobic Symptoms ... With Onset During Intoxication	← Additional differentiation in the DSM without separate codes.		*No corresponding category, code as F14.8 Other mental and behavioral disorders.*

	DSM-IV-TR	cross-walk		ICD-10
	Caffeine-Related Disorders	**Continuation**	**F15**	**Disorders Due to Use of Other Stimulants, Including Caffeine**
292.89	Caffeine-Induced Sleep Disorder ... Insomnia Type ... Hypersomnia Type ... Parasomnia Type ... Mixed Type ... With Onset During Intoxication	← Additional differentiation in the DSM without separate codes.		*No corresponding category, code as F15.8 Other mental and behavioral disorders.*
292.9	Caffeine-Related Disorder NOS	←→	F15.9	Unspecified mental and behavioral disorder
	Cocaine-Related Disorders		**F14**	**Disorders Due to Use of Cocaine**
	Cocaine Use Disorders			
304.20	Cocaine Dependence	←→	F14.2	Dependence syndrome
	With Physiological Dependence Without Physiological Dependence Early Full Remission Early Partial Remission Sustained Full Remission Sustained Partial Remission In a Controlled Environment	← Additional differentiation in the DSM without separate codes. ←→	 F14.21	*No corresponding differentiation.* Currently abstinent but in a protected environment
305.60	Cocaine Abuse	←→	F14.1	Harmful use
	Cocaine-Induced Disorders			
292.89	Cocaine Intoxication ... With Perceptual Disturbances	←→ ←→ Additional differentiation in the DSM without separate codes.	F14.0 F14.04	Acute intoxication ... With perceptional distortions
292.0	Cocaine Withdrawal	←→	F14.3	Withdrawal state
292.81	Cocaine Intoxication Delirium	←→	F14.03	Acute intoxication... With delirium
292.11 292.12 	Cocaine-Induced Psychotic Disorder ... With Delusions ... With Hallucinations ... With Onset During Intoxication	 ←→ ←→ ← Additional differentiation in the DSM without separate codes.	 F14.51 F14.52 	 Psychotic disorder ... Predominantly delusional Psychotic disorder... Predominantly hallucinatory *No corresponding differentiation.*

	DSM-IV-TR	cross-walk		ICD-10
	Cocaine-Related Disorders	**Continuation**	**F14**	**Disorders Due to Use of Cocaine**
292.84	Cocaine-Induced Mood Disorder	←		*No corresponding category, code as F14.8 Other mental and behavioral disorders, except for*
	... With Depressive Features	←→	F14.54	Psychotic disorder... Predominantly depressive symptoms
	... With Manic Features	←→	F14.55	Psychotic disorder... Predominantly manic symptoms
	... With Mixed Features	←→	F14.56	Psychotic disorder... Mixed
	... With Onset During Intoxication ... With Onset During Withdrawal	← Additional differentiation in the DSM without separate codes.		*No corresponding differentiation.*
292.89	Cocaine-Induced Anxiety Disorder ... With Generalized Anxiety ... With Panic Attacks ... With Obsessive-Compulsive Symptoms ... With Phobic Symptoms ... With Onset During Intoxication ... With Onset During Withdrawal	← Additional differentiation in the DSM without separate codes.		*No corresponding category, code as F14.8 Other mental and behavioral disorders.*
292.89	Cocaine-Induced Sexual Dysfunction ... With Impaired Desire ... With Impaired Arousal ... With Impaired Orgasm ... With Sexual Pain ... With Onset During Intoxication	← Additional differentiation in the DSM without separate codes.		*No corresponding category, code as F14.8 Other mental and behavioral disorders.*
292.89	Cocaine-Induced Sleep Disorder ... Insomnia Type ... Hypersomnia Type ... Parasomnia Type ... Mixed Type ... With Onset During Intoxication ... With Onset During Withdrawal	← Additional differentiation in the DSM without separate codes.		*No corresponding category, code as F14.8 Other mental and behavioral disorders.*
292.9	Cocaine-Related Disorder NOS	←→	F14.9	Unspecified mental and behavioral disorder

	DSM-IV-TR	cross-walk		ICD-10
	Nicotine-Related Disorders		**F17**	**Disorders Due to Use of Tobacco**
	Disorders Due to Use of Tobacco			
305.1	Nicotine Dependence	←——→	F17.2	Dependence syndrome
	With Physiological Dependence Without Physiological Dependence Early Full Remission Early Partial Remission Sustained Full Remission Sustained Partial Remission	←—— Additional differentiation in the DSM without separate codes.		*No corresponding differentiation.*
	On Agonist Therapy	←——→	F17.22	Currently on a clinically supervised mainte-nance or replacement regime
292.0	Nicotine Withdrawal	←——→	F17.3	Withdrawal state
292.9	Nicotine-Related Disorder NOS	←——→	F17.9	Unspecified mental and behavioral disorder
	Opioid-Related Disorders		**F11**	**Disorders Due To Use Of Opioids**
	Disorders Due to Use of Opioids			
304.00	Opioid Dependence	←——→	F11.2	Dependence syndrome
	With Physiological Dependence Without Physiological Dependence Early Full Remission Early Partial Remission Sustained Full Remission Sustained Partial Remission	←—— Additional differentiation in the DSM without separate codes.		*No corresponding differentiation.*
	On Agonist Therapy	←——→	F11.22	Currently on a clinically supervised mainte-nance or replacement regime
	In a Controlled Environment	←——→	F11.21	Currently abstinent but in a protected environ-ment
305.50	Opioid Abuse	←——→	F11.1	Harmful use
	Opioid-Induced Disorders			
292.89	Opioid Intoxication ... With Perceptual Disturbances	←——→ ←——→ Additional differentiation in the DSM without separate codes.	F11.0 F11.04	Acute intoxication ... With perceptional distortions
292.0	Opioid Withdrawal	←——→	F11.3	Withdrawal state
292.81	Opioid Intoxication Delirium	←——→	F11.03	Acute intoxication... With delirium

	DSM-IV-TR	cross-walk	F11	ICD-10
	Opioid-Related Disorders	Continuation		Disorders Due to Use of Opioids
	Opioid-Induced Psychotic Disorder			
292.11	... With Delusions	←——→	F11.51	Psychotic disorder ... Predominantly delusional
292.12	... With Hallucinations	←——→	F11.52	Psychotic disorder... Predominantly hallucinatory
	... With Onset During Intoxication	←—— Additional differentiation in the DSM without separate codes.		*No corresponding differentiation.*
292.84	Opioid-Induced Mood Disorder	←——		*No directly corresponding category, code as F11.8 Other mental and behavioral disorders, except for*
	... With Depressive Features	←——→	F11.54	Psychotic disorder... Predominantly depressive symptoms
	... With Manic Features	←——→	F11.55	Psychotic disorder... Predominantly manic symptoms
	... With Mixed Features	←——→	F11.56	Psychotic disorder... Mixed
	... With Onset During Intoxication	←—— Additional differentiation in the DSM without separate codes.		*No corresponding differentiation.*
292.89	Opioid-Induced Sexual Dysfunction ... With Impaired Desire ... With Impaired Arousal ... With Impaired Orgasm ... With Sexual Pain ... With Onset During Intoxication	←—— Additional differentiation in the DSM without separate codes.		*No corresponding category, code as F11.8 Other mental and behavioral disorders.*
292.89	Opioid-Induced Sleep Disorder ... Insomnia Type ... Hypersomnia Type ... Parasomnia Type ... Mixed Type ... With Onset During Intoxication ... With Onset During Withdrawal	←—— Additional differentiation in the DSM without separate codes.		*No corresponding category, code as F11.8 Other mental and behavioral disorders.*
292.9	Opioid-Induced Disorder NOS	←——→	F11.9	Unspecified mental and behavioral disorder

	DSM-IV-TR	cross-walk		ICD-10
	Phencyclidine (or Phencyclidine-Like)- Related Disorders	Phencyclidine is not coded separately in the ICD-10.	**F19**	**Disorders Due to Multiple Drug Use and Use of Other Psychoactive Substances**
	Disorder Due to Use of Phencyclidine			
304.90	Phencyclidine Dependence	←——→	F19.2	Dependence syndrome
	Early Full Remission	←——		
	Early Partial Remission			*No corresponding differentiation.*
	Sustained Full Remission	Additional differentiation in the DSM without separate codes.		
	Sustained Partial Remission			
	In a Controlled Environment	←——→	F19.21	Currently abstinent but in a protected environment
305.90	Phencyclidine Abuse	←——→	F19.1	Harmful use
	Phencyclidine-Induced Disorders			
292.89	Phencyclidine Intoxication	←——→	F19.0	Acute intoxication
	... With Perceptual Disturbances	←——→	F19.04	... With perceptional distortions
		Additional differentiation in the DSM without separate codes.		
292.81	Phencyclidine Intoxication Delirium	←——→	F19.03	Acute intoxication ... With delirium
	Phencyclidine-Induced Psychotic Disorder			
292.11	... With Delirium	←——→	F19.51	Psychotic disorder ... Predominantly delusional
292.12	... With Hallucinations	←——→	F19.52	Psychotic disorder... Predominantly hallucina-tory
	... With Onset During Intoxication	←——		
		Additional differentiation in the DSM without separate codes.		*No corresponding differentiation.*
292.84	Phencyclidine-Induced Mood Disorder	←——		*No corresponding category, code as F19.8 Other mental and behavioral disorders, except for*
	... With Depressive Features	←——→	F19.54	Psychotic disorder... Predominantly depressive symptoms
	... With Manic Features	←——→	F19.55	Psychotic disorder... Predominantly manic symptoms
	... With Mixed Features	←——→	F19.56	Psychotic disorder... Mixed
	... With Onset During Intoxication	←——		*No corresponding differentiation.*
		Additional differentiation in the DSM without separate codes.		
292.89	Phencyclidine-Induced Anxiety Disorder			
	... With Generalized Anxiety			*No corresponding category, code as F19.8 Other mental and behavioral disorders.*
	... With Panic Attacks	←——		
	... With Obsessive-Compulsive Symptoms	Additional differentiation in the DSM without separate codes.		
	... With Phobic Symptoms			
	... With Onset During Intoxication			
292.9	Phencyclidine-Related Disorder NOS	←——→	F19.9	Unspecified mental and behavioral disorder

49

	DSM-IV-TR	cross-walk		ICD-10
	Sedative-, Hypnotic- or Anxiolytic-Related Disorders		**F13**	**Disorders Due to Use of Sedatives or Hypnotics**
	Disorders Due to Use of Sedatives, Hypnotics, or Anxiolytics			
304.10	Sedative, Hypnotic, or Anxiolytic Dependence	←——→	F13.2	Dependence syndrome
	With Physiological Dependence Without Physiological Dependence Early Full Remission Early Partial Remission Sustained Full Remission Sustained Partial Remission In a Controlled Environment	←—— Additional differentiation in the DSM without separate codes. ←——→		*No corresponding differentiation.* F13.21 — Currently abstinent but in a protected environment
305.40	Sedative, Hypnotic, or Anxiolytic Abuse	←——→	F13.1	Harmful use
	Sedative-, Hypnotic- or Anxiolytic-Induced Disorders			
292.89	Sedative, Hypnotic, or Anxiolytic Intoxication	←——→	F13.0	Acute intoxication
292.0	Sedative, Hypnotic, or Anxiolytic Withdrawal ... With Perceptual Disturbances	←——→ ←—— Additional differentiation in the DSM without separate codes.	F13.3	Withdrawal state *No corresponding differentiation.*
292.81	Sedative, Hypnotic, or Anxiolytic Intoxication Delirium	←——→	F13.03	Acute intoxication ... With delirium
292.81	Sedative, Hypnotic, or Anxiolytic Withdrawal Delirium	←——→	F13.4	Withdrawal state with delirium
292.82	Sedative-, Hypnotic-, or Anxiolytic-Induced Persisting Dementia	←——→	F13.73	Residual and late-onset psychotic disorder ... Dementia
292.83	Sedative-, Hypnotic-, or Anxiolytic-Induced Persisting Amnestic Disorder	←——→	F13.6	Amnesic syndrome
292.11 292.12	Sedative-, Hypnotic-, or Anxiolytic-Induced Psychotic Disorder ... With Delusions ... With Hallucinations ... With Onset During Intoxication ... With Onset During Withdrawal	 ←——→ ←——→ ←—— Additional differentiation in the DSM without separate codes.	F13.51 F13.52	 Psychotic disorder... Predominantly delusional Psychotic disorder... Predominantly hallucinatory *No corresponding differentiation.*

	DSM-IV-TR	cross-walk	ICD-10	
	Sedative-, Hypnotic-, or Anxiolytic-Related Disorders	**Continuation**	**F13**	**Disorders Due to Use of Sedatives or Hypnotics**
292.84	Sedative-, Hypnotic-, or Anxiolytic-Induced Mood Disorder	←	*No corresponding category, code as F13.8 Other mental and behavioral disorders, except for*	
	... With Depressive Features	←→	F13.54	Psychotic disorder... Predominantly depressive Symptoms
	... With Manic Features	←→	F13.55	Psychotic disorder... Predominantly manic Symptoms
	... With Mixed Features	←→	F13.56	Psychotic disorder... Mixed
	... With Onset During Intoxication ... With Onset During Withdrawal	← Additional differentiation in the DSM without separate codes.	*No corresponding differentiation.*	
292.89	Sedative-, Hypnotic-, or Anxiolytic-Induced Anxiety Disorder ... With Generalized Anxiety ... With Panic Attacks ... With Obsessive-Compulsive Symptoms ... With Phobic Symptoms ... With Onset During Withdrawal	← Additional differentiation in the DSM without separate codes.	*No corresponding category, code as F13.8 Other mental and behavioral disorders.*	
292.89	Sedative-, Hypnotic-, or Anxiolytic-Induced Sexual Dysfunction ... With Impaired Desire ... With Impaired Arousal ... With Impaired Orgasm ... With Sexual Pain ... With Onset During Intoxication	← Additional differentiation in the DSM without separate codes.	*No corresponding category, code as F13.8 Other mental and behavioral disorders.*	
292.89	Sedative-, Hypnotic-, or Anxiolytic-Induced Sleep Disorder ... Insomnia Type ... Hypersomnia Type ... Parasomnia Type ... Mixed Type ... With Onset During Intoxication ... With Onset During Withdrawal	← Additional differentiation in the DSM without separate codes.	*No corresponding category, code as F13.8 Other mental and behavioral disorders.*	
292.9	Sedative-, Hypnotic-, or Anxiolytic-Related Disorder NOS	←→	F13.9	Unspecified mental and behavioral disorder
	Polysubstance-Related Disorders			
304.80	Polysubstance Dependence	←→	F19.2	Disorders due to multiple drug use and use of other psychoactive substances ... Dependence syndrome

51

	DSM-IV-TR	cross-walk		ICD-10
	Other (or Unknown) Substance-Related Disorders		**F19**	**Disorders Due to Multiple Drug Use and Use of Other Psychoactive Substances**
	Other (or Unknown) Substance Use Disorders			
304.90	Other (or Unknown) Substance Dependence	◄──►	F19.2	Dependence syndrome
	With Physiological Dependence Without Physiological Dependence Early Full Remission Early Partial Remission Sustained Full Remission Sustained Partial Remission On Agonist Therapy In a Controlled Environment	◄── Additional differentiation in the DSM without separate codes. ◄──► ◄──►	 F19.22 F19.21	*No corresponding differentiation.* Currently on a clinically supervised maintenance or replacement regime Currently abstinent but in a protected environment
305.90	Other (or Unknown) Substance Abuse		F19.1	Harmful use
	Other (or Unknown) Substance-Related Disorders			
292.89	Other (or Unknown) Substance Intoxication ... With Perceptual Disturbances	◄──► ◄──► Additional differentiation in the DSM without separate codes.	F19.0 F19.04	Acute intoxication ... With perceptional distortions
292.0	Other (or Unknown) Substance Withdrawal ... With Perceptual Disturbances	◄──► ◄── Additional differentiation in the DSM without separate codes.	F19.3	Withdrawal state *No corresponding differentiation.*
292.81	Other (or Unknown) Substance-Induced Delirium	◄──►	F19.03	Acute intoxication ... With delirium
292.82	Other (or Unknown) Substance-Induced Persisting Dementia	◄──►	F19.73	Residual and late-onset psychotic disorder ... Dementia
292.83	Other (or Unknown) Substance-Induced Persisting Amnestic Disorder	◄──►	F19.6	Amnesic syndrome

	DSM-IV-TR	cross-walk		ICD-10
	Other (or Unknown) Substance-Related Disorders	**Continuation**		**Disorders Due to (Multiple Drug Use and) Use of Other Psychoactive Substances**
292.11 292.12	Other (or Unknown) Substance-Induced Psychotic Disorder ... With Delusions ... With Hallucinations ... With Onset During Intoxication ... With Onset During Withdrawal	←——→ ←——→ ←—— *Additional differentiation in the DSM without separate codes.*	F19.51 F19.52	Psychotic Disorder ... Predominantly delusional Psychotic Disorder... Predominantly hallucinatory *No corresponding differentiation.*
292.84	Other (or Unknown) Substance-Induced Mood Disorder ... With Depressive Features ... With Manic Features ... With Mixed Features ... With Onset During Intoxication ... With Onset During Withdrawal	←—— ←——→ ←——→ ←——→ ←—— *Additional differentiation in the DSM without separate codes.*	F19.54 F19.55 F19.56	*No directly corresponding category, code as F19.8 Other mental and behavioral disorder, except for* Psychotic disorder... Predominantly depressive symptoms Psychotic disorder... Predominantly manic symptoms Psychotic disorder... Mixed *No corresponding differentiation.*
292.89	Other (or Unknown) Substance-Induced Anxiety Disorder ... With Generalized Anxiety ... With Panic Attacks ... With Obsessive-Compulsive Symptoms ... With Phobic Symptoms ... With Onset During Withdrawal	←—— *Additional differentiation in the DSM without separate codes.*		*No corresponding category, code as F19.8 Other mental and behavioral disorders.*
292.89	Other (or Unknown) Substance-Induced Sexual Dysfunction ... With Impaired Desire ... With Impaired Arousal ... With Impaired Orgasm ... With Sexual Pain ... With Onset During Intoxication	←—— *Additional differentiation in the DSM without separate codes.*		*No corresponding category, code as F19.8 Other mental and behavioral disorders.*
292.89	Other (or Unknown) Substance-Induced Sleep Disorder ... Insomnia Type ... Hypersomnia Type ... Parasomnia Type ... Mixed Type ... With Onset During Intoxication ... With Onset During Withdrawal	←—— *Additional differentiation in the DSM without separate codes.*		*No corresponding category, code as F19.8 Other mental and behavioral disorders.*
292.9	Other (or Unknown) Substance-Related Disorder NOS	←——→	F19.9	*Unspecified mental and behavioral disorder*

	DSM-IV-TR	cross-walk		ICD-10
	Schizophrenia and Other Psychotic Disorders		**F2**	**Schizophrenia, Schizotypal and Delusional Disorders**
295.xx	**Schizophrenia**	Observation period in the DSM > 6 months.	**F20**	**Schizophrenia**
	Differentiation of patterns of course without separate code in the DSM, for all schizophrenia types:			The coding of patterns of course takes place at the 5th position of the ICD-10:
	Episodic With Interepisode Residual Symptoms	←		*5th Position is not to be coded if it is impossible to definitely relate to* *F20.x1 Episodic with progressive deficit or* *F20.x2 Episodic with stable deficit.*
	Episodic With No Interepisode Residual Symptoms	←→	F20.x3	Episodic remittent
	Continuous	←→	F20.x0	Continuous
	Single Episode In Partial Remission	←→	F20.x4	Incomplete remission
	Single Episode In Full Remission	←→	F20.x5	Complete remission
	Other or Unspecified Pattern	←→	F20.x8	Other pattern of course
	Determine if the Residual symptoms are ... With Prominent Negative Symptoms	←		*No corresponding differentiation.*
295.3	Paranoid Type	←→	F20.0	Paranoid schizophrenia
295.10	Disorganized Type	←→	F20.1	Hebephrenic schizophrenia
295.20	Catatonic Type	←→ Symptoms in the ICD ≥ 2 weeks.	F20.2	Catatonic schizophrenia
295.90	Undifferentiated Type	←→	F20.3	Undifferentiated schizophrenia
295.60	Residual Type	←→	F20.5	Residual schizophrenia
295.40	Schizophreniform Disorder ... With / Without Good Prognostic Features	← Symptoms >1 month and < 6 months. Additional differentiation in the DSM without separate codes.		*No corresponding category, code as F20.8 Other schizophrenia (not F23.1 Acute polymorphic psychotic disorder with symptoms of schizophrenia, or F23.2 Acute schizophrenia-like psychotic disorder).*
295.70	Schizoaffective Disorder Bipolar Type Depressive Type	← Additional differentiation in the DSM without separate codes.		*If impossible to definitely relate to* *F25.0 Schizoaffective disorder, manic type or* *F25.2 Schizoaffective disorder, mixed type* *code as F25.9 Schizoaffective disorder, unspecified.*
		←→	F25.1	Schizoaffective disorder, depressive type

	DSM-IV-TR	cross-walk	F2	ICD-10
	Schizophrenia and Other Psychotic Disorders	**Continuation**		**Schizophrenia, Schizotypal and Delusional Disorders**
297.1	Delusional Disorder	←→ Symptoms in the DSM > 1 month, in the ICD-10 > 3 months. Respective disorders of < 3 months are coded in the ICD-10 among F23.	F22.0	Delusional disorder
	Erotomanic Type Grandiose Type Jealous Type Persecutory Type Somatic Type Mixed Type Unspecified Type	← Additional differentiation in the DSM without separate codes.		*No corresponding differentiation.*
	Psychotic Disorders			
298.8	Brief Psychotic Disorder	← Symptoms in the ICD-10 < 3 months, for F23.1 and F23.2 < 1 month (for differentiation from F20 Schizophrenia). In the DSM symptoms generally < 1 month, otherwise code as 297.1 Delusional Disorder.		*Additional differentiation based on the predominant symptoms in the ICD-10, therefore code as F23.9 Acute and transient psychotic disorder, unspecified.*
	Without Marked Stressors With Marked Stressors With Postpartum Onset	←→ ←→ ← Additional differentiation in the DSM without separate codes.	F23.90 F23.91	With symptoms of schizophrenia Without symptoms of schizophrenia *No corresponding category.*
297.3	Shared Psychotic Disorder	←→	F24	Induced delusional disorder
	Psychotic Disorder Due to... *[Indicate the General Medical Condition]*			
293.81	With Delusions	←→	F06.2	Organic delusional (schizophrenia-like) disorder
293.82	With Hallucinations	←→	F06.0	Organic hallucinosis
—.-	*Substance-Induced Psychotic Disorder (for substance-specific codes refer to Substance-Related Disorders)*	←→		
298.9	Psychotic Disorder NOS	←→	F29	Unspecified nonorganic psychosis

	DSM-IV-TR	cross-walk		ICD-10
	Mood Disorders		**F3**	**Mood (Affective) Disorders**
	Depressive Disorders			
	Major Depression, Single Episode			**Depressive Episodes**
	Chronic With Catatonic Features With Melancholic Features With Atypical Features With Postpartum Onset	← Additional differentiation in the DSM without separate codes.		*No corresponding differentiation.*
296.21	Mild	←→	F32.0	Mild depressive episode
296.22	Moderate	←→	F32.1	Moderate depressive episode

296.23
296.24
	Severe
	    Without Psychotic Features
	    With Psychotic Features
		←→
		←→
			F32.2
			F32.3
				Severe depressive episode
				    Without psychotic symptoms
				    With psychotic symptoms

	... Mood-Congruent ... Mood-Incongruent	← Additional differentiation in the DSM without separate codes.		*No corresponding differentiation.*
296.25	In Partial Remission			*No corresponding category, code as F32.9 Depressive episode, unspecified.*
296.26	In Full Remission	←		
296.20	Unspecified			
296.3	**Major Depression, Recurrent**			**Recurrent Depressive Disorder**
	Chronic With Catatonic Features With Melancholic Features With Atypical Features With Postpartum Onset With/Without Interepisode Recovery With Seasonal Pattern	← Additional differentiation in the DSM without separate codes.		*No corresponding differentiation.*
296.31	Mild	←→	F33.0	Current episode mild
296.32	Moderate	←→	F33.1	Current Episode Moderate

296.33
296.34
	Severe
	    Without Psychotic Features
	    With Psychotic Features
		←→
		←→
			F33.2
			F33.3
				Current Episode Severe
				    Without Psychotic Symptoms
				    With Psychotic Symptoms

	... Mood-Congruent ... Mood-Incongruent	← Additional differentiation in the DSM without separate codes.		*No corresponding differentiation.*
296.35	In Partial Remission	←		*No corresponding category, code as F33.9 Recurrent depressive disorder, unspecified.*

DSM-IV-TR		cross-walk		ICD-10	
Depressive Disorders		**Continuation**			
296.36	In Full Remission	←——→	F33.4	Recurrent depressive disorder, currently in remission	
296.30	Unspecified	←——		*No corresponding category, code as F33.9 Recurrent depressive disorder, unspecified..*	
300.4	Dysthymic Disorder	←——→	F34.1	Dysthymia	
	Early Onset	←——			
	Late Onset	Additional differentiation in the DSM without separate codes.		*No corresponding differentiation.*	
	With Atypical Features				
311	Depressive Disorder NOS	——→	F32.9	Depressive episode, unspecified.	
Bipolar Disorders				**Bipolar Affective Disorders**	
Bipolar I Disorders					
296.0x	Single Manic Episode		F30	Manic episode	
	Mixed	←——		*No corresponding differentiation.*	
	With Catatonic Features	Additional differentiation in the DSM without separate codes.			
	With Postpartum Onset				
296.01	Mild				
296.02	Moderate	←——		*No directly corresponding category, code as F30.1 Mania without psychotic symptoms.*	
296.03	Severe	No differentiation on severity in the ICD-10.			
	Without Psychotic Features				
296.04	With Psychotic Features	←——→	F30.2	Mania with psychotic symptoms	
	... Mood-Congruent	←——→	F30.20	... Mood-Congruent	
	... Mood-Incongruent	←——→	F30.21	... Mood-Incongruent	
		Additional differentiation in the DSM without separate codes.			
296.05	In Partial Remission			*No corresponding category, code as F30.9 Manic episode, unspecified.*	
296.06	In Full Remission	←——			
296.00	Unspecified				
296.40	Most Recent Episode Hypomanic	←——→	F31.0	Bipolar affective disorder, current episode hypomanic	
	With/Without Interepisode Recovery	←——			
	With Seasonal Pattern	Additional differentiation in the DSM without separate codes.		*No corresponding differentiation.*	
	With Rapid Cycling				

	DSM-IV-TR	cross-walk		ICD-10
	Bipolar I Disorders	**Continuation**		**Bipolar Affective Disorders**
296.4x	Most Recent Episode Manic			Current episode manic
	Chronic With Catatonic Features With Melancholic Features With Atypical Features With Postpartum Onset With/Without Interepisode Recovery With Rapid Cycling	← Additional differentiation in the DSM without separate codes.		*No corresponding differentiation.*
296.41	Mild			*No directly corresponding category, code as F31.1 ... Current episode manic without psychotic symptoms.*
296.42	Moderate	←		
296.43	Severe Without Psychotic Features	No differentiation on severity in the ICD-10.		
296.44	With Psychotic Features ... Mood-Congruent ... Mood-Incongruent	←→ ←→ ←→ Additional differentiation in the DSM without separate codes.	F31.2 F31.20 F31.21	With psychotic symptoms Mood-congruent Mood-incongruent
296.45	In Partial Remission			*No corresponding category, code as F31.9 Bipolar affective disorder, unspecified. For 296.46 consider also F31.7 Bipolar affective disorder, currently in remission.*
296.46	In Full Remission	←		
296.40	Unspecified			
296.6x	Most Recent Episode Mixed			
	With Catatonic Features With Postpartum Onset With/Without Interepisode Recovery With Seasonal Pattern With Rapid Cycling	← Additional differentiation in the DSM without separate codes.		
296.61	Mild			
296.62	Moderate	←		
296.63	Severe Without Psychotic Features			*No corresponding differentiation, code as F31.6 Bipolar affective disorder, current episode mixed.*
296.64	With Psychotic Features ... Mood-Congruent ... Mood-Incongruent	← Additional differentiation in the DSM without separate codes.		

	DSM-IV-TR	cross-walk		ICD-10
	Bipolar I Disorders	**Continuation**		**Bipolar Affective Disorders**
296.65	In Partial Remission			*No corresponding differentiation, code as*
296.66	In Full Remission	←		*F31.6 Bipolar affective disorder, current episode mixed.*
296.60	Unspecified			
296.5x	Most Recent Episode Depressed			Current episode depression
	Chronic With Catatonic Features With Melancholic Features With Atypical Features With Postpartum Onset With/Without Interepisode Recovery With Seasonal Pattern With Rapid Cycling	← Additional differentiation in the DSM without separate codes		*No corresponding differentiation.*
296.51	Mild	←→	F31.1	Moderate or mild
296.52	Moderate			
296.53	Severe Without Psychotic Features		F31.4	Severe without psychotic symptoms
296.54	With Psychotic Features ... Mood-Congruent ... Mood-Incongruent	←→ ←→ ←→ Additional differentiation in the DSM without separate codes.	F31.5 F31.50 F31.51	Severe with psychotic symptoms Mood-congruent Mood-incongruent
296.55	In Partial Remission			*No corresponding category, code as F31.9 Bipolar affective*
296.56	In Full Remission	←		*disorder, unspecified. For 296.56 consider also F31.7 Bipolar affective disorder, currently in remission..*
296.50	Unspecified			
296.7	Most Recent Episode Unspecified			
	With/Without Interepisode Recovery	←		
	With Seasonal Pattern	Additional differentiation in the DSM without separate codes.		*No corresponding category, code as F31.9 Bipolar affective disorder, unspecified.*
	With Rapid Cycling			

	DSM-IV-TR	cross-walk		ICD-10
	Bipolar Disorders			**Bipolar Affective Disorders**
296.89	Bipolar II Disorders	←		*No directly corresponding category, code as F31.9 Bipolar affective disorder, unspecified.*
	Chronic With Catatonic Features With Melancholic Features With Atypical Features With Postpartum Onset With/Without Interepisode Recovery With Seasonal Pattern (only applies to Major Depressive Episode) With Rapid Cycling			
	Current (or Most Recent) Episode Hypomanic	←		

	Current (or Most Recent) Episode
	Depressed
	  Mild
	  Moderate
	  Severe
	    ... Without Psychotic Features
	    ... With Psychotic Features
	    ... Mood-Congruent
	    ... Mood-Incongruent
	  In Partial Remission
	  In Full Remission
	  Unspecified
		Differentiation in the DSM without separate codes.		*No corresponding category, for hypomanic episode code F31.0 ... Current episode hypomanic and for depressive episode F31.8 Other bipolar affective disorders.*

301.13	Cyclothymic Disorder	←→	F34.0	Cyclothymia
296.80	Bipolar Disorder NOS	←→	F31.9	Bipolar affective disorder, unspecified
293.83	Mood Disorder Due to ... *[Indicate the General Medical Condition]*			
	With Depressive Features With Major-Depressive-Like Episode	←→ Differentiation in the DSM without separate codes.	F06.32	Organic depressive disorder
	With Manic Features With Mixed Features	←→ ←→	F06.30 F06.33	Organic manic disorder Organic mixed affective disorder
--.-	*Substance-Induced Mood Disorder (for substance-specific codes refer to Substance-Related Disorders)*	←→	--.-	
296.90	Mood Disorder NOS		F39	Unspecified mood (affective) disorder

	DSM-IV-TR	cross-walk	In: F4	ICD-10
	Anxiety Disorders		**In: F4**	**Neurotic, Stress-Related and Somatoform Disorders**
300.01	Panic Disorder Without Agoraphobia	←→	F41.0	Panic disorder (episodic paroxysmal anxiety)
300.21	Panic Disorder With Agoraphobia	←→	F40.01	Agoraphobia with panic disorder
300.22	Agoraphobia Without History of Panic Disorder	←→	F40.00	Agoraphobia without panic disorder

300.29	Specific Phobia
	    Animal Type
	    Natural Environment Type
	    Blood-Injection-Injury-Type
	    Situational Type
	    Other Type
		←→
		
		←
		Additional differentiation in the DSM without separate codes.
			F40.2	Specific (isolated) phobias
				
				No corresponding differentiation.

300.23	Social Phobia Generalized	←→ ← Additional differentiation in the DSM without separate codes.	F40.1	Social phobias *No corresponding differentiation.*
300.3	Obsessive-Compulsive Disorder With Poor Insight	←→ ← Additional differentiation in the DSM without separate codes.	F42.9	Obsessive-compulsive disorder, unspecified *No corresponding differentiation*

309.81	Posttraumatic Stress Disorder
	    Acute/Chronic
	    Chronic
	    With Delayed Onset
		←→
		In the DSM ≥1 month
		←
		Additional differentiation in the DSM without separate codes.
			F43.1	Post-traumatic stress disorder
				
				No corresponding differentiation.

308.3	Acute Stress Disorder	←→ In the ICD-10 onset after <1 hour, diminishing after 8-48 h.	F43.0	Acute stress reaction
300.02	Generalized Anxiety Disorder	←→	F41.1	Generalized anxiety disorder

293.84	Anxiety Disorder Due to ...
	[Indicate the General Medical Condition]
	    With Generalized Anxiety
	    With Panic Attacks
	    With Obsessive-Compulsive Symptoms
		←→
		
		←
		Additional differentiation in the DSM without separate codes.
			F06.4	Organic anxiety disorder
				
				No corresponding differentiation.

--.-	*Substance-Induced Anxiety Disorder (for substance-specific codes refer to Substance-Related Disorders)*		--.-	
300.00	Anxiety Disorder NOS	←→	F41.9	Anxiety disorder, unspecified

DSM-IV-TR		cross-walk		ICD-10	
Somatoform Disorders				**Somatoform Disorders**	
300.81	Somatization Disorder	←——→ *In the ICD-10 Symptoms ≥ 2 years, in the DSM "several years".*	F45.0	Somatization disorder	
300.82	Somatoform Disorder NOS	←——→	F45.1	Undifferentiated somatoform disorder *Consider also F68.0 Elaboration of physical symptoms for psychological reasons*	
300.11	Conversion Disorder			*No directly corresponding category, if impossible to relate to any differentiation code as F44.9 Dissociative (conversion) disorder, unspecified.*	
	With Motor Symptom or Deficit	←——		*No corresponding differentiation.*	
	With Sensory Symptom or Deficit	←——→	F44.6	Dissociative anaesthesia and sensory loss	
	With Seizures or Convulsions	←——→	F44.5	Dissociative convulsions	
	With Mixed Presentation	←——→ *Additional differentiation in the DSM without separate codes.*	F44.7	Mixed dissociative (conversion) disorders	
307.8x	Pain Disorder ... Acute: < 6 months ... Chronic: > 6 months	←—— *Additional differentiation in the DSM without separate codes.*		*No corresponding differentiation.*	
307.80	Pain Disorder Associated With Psychological Factors	←——→ *Differentiation not available in the ICD-10.*	F45.4	Persistent somatoform pain disorder *(If necessary, code the additional illness)*	
307.89	Pain Disorder Associated With Both Psychological Factors and a General Medical Condition				
300.7	Hypochondriasis With Poor Insight	←——→ ←—— *Additional differentiation in the DSM without separate codes.*	F45.2	Hypochondriacal disorder *No corresponding differentiation.*	
300.7	Body Dysmorphic Disorder	←——		*No corresponding category, code as F45.2 Hypochondriacal disorder*	
300.82	Somatoform Disorder NOS	←——→	F45.9	Somatoform disorder, unspecified	
Factitious Disorders					
300.16	With Predominantly Psychological Signs and Symptoms	←——→ *Differentiation not available in the ICD-10.*	F68.1	Intentional production or feigning of symptoms or disabilities, either physical or psychological (factitious disorder)	
300.19	With Predominantly Physical Signs and Symptoms				

	DSM-IV-TR	cross-walk		ICD-10
	Factitious Disorders	**Continuation**		
300.19	With Combined Psychological and Physical Signs and Symptoms	←——→ Differentiation not available in the ICD-10.	F68.1	Intentional production or feigning of symptoms or disabilities, either physical or psychological (factitious disorder)
300.19	Factitious Disorder NOS			
	Dissociative Disorders			**Dissociative Disorders**
300.12	Dissociative Amnesia	←——→	F44.0	Dissociative amnesia
300.13	Dissociative Fugue	←——→	F44.1	Dissociative fugue
300.14	Dissociative Identity Disorder	←——→	F44.81	Multiple personality disorder
300.6	Depersonalization Disorder	←——→	F48.1	Depersonalization-derealization syndrome
300.15	Dissociative Disorder NOS	←——→	F44.9	Dissociative (conversion) disorder, unspecified
	Sexual and Gender Identity Disorders	In the ICD-10 symptoms ≥ 6 months.	**F52**	**Sexual Dysfunction, Not Caused By Organic Disorder or Disease**
	Sexual Dysfunctions			
	Lifelong Type Acquired Type Generalized Type Situational Type Due to Psychological Factors Due to Combined Factors	←—— Additional differentiation in the DSM without separate codes.		*No corresponding differentiation.*
302.71 302.79	Sexual Desire Disorders Hypoactive Sexual Desire Disorder Sexual Aversion Disorder	←——→ ←——→	F52.0 F52.10	Lack or loss or sexual desire Sexual aversion
302.72 302.72	Sexual Arousal Disorder Female Sexual Arousal Disorder Male Erectile Disorder	←——→ Differentiation not available in the ICD-10.	F52.2	Failure of genital response
302.73 302.74	Orgasmic Disorders Female Orgasmic Disorder Male Orgasmic Disorder	←——→ Differentiation not available in the ICD-10.	F52.3	Orgasmic dysfunction
302.75	Premature Ejaculation	←——→	F52.4	Premature ejaculation
302.76 306.51	Sexual Pain Disorders Dyspareunia (Not Due to a Medical Condition) Vaginismus (Not Due to a Medical Condition)	←——→ ←——→	F52.6 F52.5	Nonorganic dyspareunia Nonorganic vaginismus

	DSM-IV-TR	cross-walk		ICD-10
	Sexual and Gender Identity Disorders	**Continuation**		**Sexual Dysfunction, Not Caused By Organic Disorder or Disease**
	Sexual Dysfunction Due to... [Indicate the General Medical Condition]	←		*No corresponding category, code as F06.8 Other specified mental disorder due to brain damage and dysfunction and to physical disease plus additional diagnosis (N – Diseases of the genitourinary system).*
625.8	Female Hypoactive Sexual Desire Disorder Due to ...			*Additional diagnose N94.8*
608.89	Male Hypoactive Sexual Desire Disorder Due to...			*Additional diagnose N50.8*
607.84	Male Erectile Disorder Due to ...	←		*Additional diagnose N48.4*
625.0	Female Dyspareunia Due to...			*Additional diagnose N94.1*
608.89	Male Dyspareunia Due to...			*Additional diagnose N50.8*
625.8	Other Female Sexual dysfunction Due to...			*Additional diagnose N94.8*
608.89	Other Male Sexual dysfunction Due to...			*Additional diagnose N50.8*
--.-	*Substance-Induced Sexual Dysfunction (for substance-specific codes refer to Substance-Related Disorders)*		--.-	
302.70	Sexual Dysfunction NOS	←→	F52.9	Unspecified sexual dysfunction, not caused by organic disorder or disease
Paraphilias			**F65**	**Disorders of Sexual Preference**
302.4	Exhibitionism	←→	F65.2	Exhibitionism
302.81	Fetishism	←→	F65.0	Fetishism
302.89	Frotteurism	←→		*No corresponding category, code as F65.8 Other disorders of sexual preference.*
302.2	Pedophilia Sexually Attracted to Males Sexually Attracted to Females Sexually Attracted to Both Limited to Incest Exclusive Type Nonexclusive Type	← *Additional differentiation in the DSM without separate codes.*	F65.4 *No corresponding differentiation.*	Paedophilia
302.83	Sexual Masochism	←→	F65.5	Sadomasochism
302.84	Sexual Sadism	*Differentiation not available in the ICD-10.*		

	DSM-IV-TR	cross-walk		ICD-10
	Paraphilias	**Continuation**	**F65**	**Disorders of Sexual Preference**
302.3	Transvestic Fetishism With Gender Dysphoria	←→ ← Additional differentiation in the DSM without separate codes.	F65.1	Fetishistic Transvestism *No corresponding differentiation.*
302.82	Voyeurism	←→	F65.3	Voyeurism
302.9	Paraphilia NOS	←→	F65.9	Disorder of sexual preference, unspecified
	Gender Identity Disorders		**F64**	**Gender Identity Disorders**
302.6	In Children	←→	F64.2	Gender identity disorder of childhood
302.85	In Adolescents or Adults	←→	F64.0	Transsexualism
	Sexually Attracted to Males Sexually Attracted to Females Sexually Attracted to Both Sexually Attracted to Neither	← Additional differentiation in the DSM without separate codes.		*No corresponding differentiation.*
302.6	Gender Identity Disorder NOS	←→	F64.9	Gender identity disorder, unspecified
302.9	Sexual Disorder NOS	←→	F52.9	Unspecified sexual dysfunction, not caused by organic disorder or disease
	Eating Disorders		**F50**	**Eating Disorders**
307.1	Anorexia nervosa	←→	F50.0	Anorexia Nervosa,
	Restrictive Type	←→	F50.00	... Without active measures for loss of weight (Vomiting, Laxatives, etc.)
	"Binge-Eating/Purging"-Type	←→ Additional differentiation in the DSM without separate codes.	F50.01	... With active measures for loss of weight (Vomiting, Laxatives, etc.)
307.51	Bulimia nervosa	←→	F50.2	Bulimia Nervosa
	"Purging"-Type "Non-Purging"-Type	← Additional differentiation in the DSM without separate codes.		*No corresponding differentiation.*
307.50	Eating Disorder NOS	←→	F50.9	Eating disorder, unspecified

	DSM-IV-TR		cross-walk			ICD-10
	Sleep Disorders				**F51**	**Nonorganic Sleep Disorders**
	Primary Sleep Disorders					
	Dyssomnias					
307.42	Primary Insomnia		←——→		F51.0	Nonorganic insomnia
307.44	Primary Hypersomnia Recurrent		←——→ ←——		F51.1	Nonorganic hypersomnia
			Additional differentiation in the DSM without separate codes.			*No corresponding differentiation.*
347	Narcolepsy		←——→		G47.4	Narcolepsy and cataplexy
780.59	Breathing-Related Sleep Disorder		←——→		G47.3	Sleep apnoea

307.45	Circadian Rhythm Sleep Disorder
	    Delayed Sleep Phase Type
	    Jet Lag Type
	    Shift Work Type
	    Unspecified Type
			←——→
			←——
			
			Additional differentiation in the DSM without separate codes.
					F51.2	Nonorganic disorder of the sleep-wake schedule
						No corresponding differentiation.

307.47	Dyssomnia NOS		←——→		F51.9	Nonorganic sleep disorder, unspecified
	Parasomnias					
307.47	Nightmare Disorder		←——→		F51.5	Nightmares
307.46	Sleep Terror Disorder		←——→		F51.4	Sleep terrors (night terrors)
307.46	Sleepwalking Disorder		←——→		F51.3	Sleepwalking (somnambulism)
307.47	Parasomnia NOS		←——			*No directly corresponding category, code as F51.8 Other nonorganic sleep disorders.*
	Sleep Disorders Related to another Mental Disorder					
307.42	Insomnia Related to... [Indicate the Axis I or Axis II Disorder]		←——			*No corresponding category, code as F51.0 Nonorganic insomnia.*
307.44	Hypersomnia Related to... [Indicate the Axis I or Axis II Disorder]		←——			*No corresponding category, code as F51.1 Nonorganic hypersomnia.*

DSM-IV-TR		cross-walk		ICD-10	
Sleep Disorders		**Continuation**	**F51**	**Nonorganic Sleep Disorders**	
Other Sleep Disorders					
780.xx	Sleep Disorder Due to... **[Indicate the General Medical Condition]**	←		**No directly corresponding category, code as F06.8 Other Specified Mental Disorder Due to Brain Damage and Dysfunction and to Physical Disease** plus additional diagnosis (G –Diseases of the nervous system).	
780.52	Insomnia-Type			***Additional diagnosis G47.0***	
780.54	Hypersomnia-Type			***Additional diagnosis G47.1***	
780.59	Parasomnia-Type			*Additional diagnosis G47.8*	
780.59	Mixed Type			***Additional diagnosis G47.8***	
--.-	*Substance-Induced Sleep Disorder (for substance-specific codes refer to Substance-Related Disorders)*		--.-		
Impulse-Control Disorders, Not Elsewhere Classified		In the ICD-10 ≥ 2 episodes within 12 months.	**F63**	**Habit and Impulse Disorders**	
312.34	Intermittent Explosive Disorder	←		*No directly corresponding category, code as F63.8 Other habit and impulse disorders.*	
312.32	Kleptomania	←→	F63.2	Pathological stealing (kleptomania)	
312.33	Pyromania	←→	F63.1	Pathological fire-setting (pyromania)	
312.31	Pathological Gambling	←→	F63.0	Pathological gambling	
312.39	Trichotillomania	←→	F63.3	Trichotillomania	
312.30	Impulse-Control Disorder NOS	←→	F63.9	Habit and impulse disorder, unspecified	
Adjustment Disorders			**F43**	**(Reaction to severe stress, and) Adjustment Disorders**	
	... Acute ... Chronic	← Additional differentiation in the DSM without separate codes.		*No corresponding differentiation.*	
309.0	With Depressed Mood	←→	F43.20	Brief depressive reaction (< 1 month)	
			F43.21	Prolonged depressive reaction (< 2 years)	
309.24	With Anxiety	←		*No directly corresponding category, code as F43.28 With other specified predominant symptoms.*	
309.28	With Mixed Anxiety and Depressed Mood	←→	F43.22	Mixed anxiety and depressive reaction	

DSM-IV-TR		cross-walk		ICD-10	
Adjustment Disorders		**continuation**	**F43**	(Reaction to severe stress, and) **Adjustment Disorders**	
309.3	With Disturbance of Conduct	←→	F43.24	With predominant disturbance of conduct	
309.4	With Mixed Disturbance of Emotions and Conduct	←→	F43.25	With mixed disturbance of emotions and conduct	
309.9	Unspecified	←→	F43.9	Reaction to severe stress, unspecified	
Personality Disorders			**F60**	**Specific Personality Disorders**	
	Cluster A- Personality Disorders				
301.0	Paranoid Personality Disorder	←→	F60.0	Paranoid personality disorder	
301.20	Schizoid Personality Disorder	←→	F60.1	Schizoid personality disorder	
301.22	Schizotypal Personality Disorder	←		*No directly corresponding category, code as F21 Schizotypal disorders.*	
	Cluster B- Personality Disorders				
301.7	Antisocial Personality Disorder	←→	F60.2	Dissocial personality disorder	
301.83	Borderline Personality Disorder	←→	F60.31	Emotionally unstable personality disorder, Borderline type	
301.50	Histrionic Personality Disorder	←→	F60.4	Histrionic personality disorder	
301.81	Narcissistic Personality Disorder	←		*No directly corresponding category, code as F60.8 Other specific personality disorder.*	
	Cluster C- Personality Disorders				
301.82	Avoidant Personality Disorder	←→	F60.6	Anxious (avoidant) personality disorder	
301.6	Dependent Personality Disorder	←→	F60.7	Dependent personality disorder	
301.4	Obsessive-Compulsive Personality Disorder	←→	F60.5	Anankastic personality disorder	
301.9	Personality Disorder NOS	←→	F60.9	Personality disorder, unspecified	

	DSM-IV-TR	cross-walk	ICD-10	
	Other Clinically Relevant Problems			
	Psychological Factors affecting a General Medical Condition		**F54**	**Psychological and Behavioral Factors Associated With Disorders or Diseases Classified Elsewhere**
316	... Specified Psychological Factor] Affecting... [Indicate the General Medical Condition]	⟷	F54	Psychological and behavioral factors associated with disorders or diseases classified elsewhere
	Mental Disorder Affecting...			
	Psychological Symptoms Affecting...			
	Personality Traits or Coping Style Affecting...	⟵ Additional differentiation in the DSM without separate codes.	*No corresponding differentiation.*	
	Maladaptive Health Behaviors Affecting...			
	Stress-Related Physiological Response Affecting...			
	Other or Unspecified Factors Affecting...			
	Medication-Induced Movement Disorders			
332.1	Neuroleptic-Induced Parkinsonism	⟵	*No directly corresponding category, code as G21.1 Other drug-induced secondary parkinsonism.*	
333.92	Neuroleptic Malignant Syndrome	⟷	G21.0	Malignant neuroleptic syndrome
333.7	Neuroleptic-Induced Acute Dystonia	⟵	*No directly corresponding category, code as G24.0 Drug-induced dystonia and dyskinesia.*	
333.99	Neuroleptic-Induced Acute Akathisia	⟵	*No directly corresponding category, code as G21.1 Other drug-induced secondary parkinsonism.*	
333.82	Neuroleptic-Induced Tardive Dyskinesia	⟵	*No directly corresponding category, code as G24.0 Drug-induced dystonia and dyskinesia.*	
333.1	Medication-Induced Postural Tremor	⟷	G25.1	Drug-induced tremor
333.90	Medication-Induced Movement Disorder NOS	⟵	*No directly corresponding category, code most likely as G25.9 Extrapyramidal and movement disorder, unspecified.*	
	Other Medication-Induced Disorders			
995.2	Adverse Effects of Medication NOS	⟷	T88.7	Unspecified adverse effect of drug or medicament

	DSM-IV-TR	cross-walk		ICD-10
Relational Problems				
V61.9	Relational Problem Related to a Mental Disorder or General Medical Condition	←		*No directly corresponding category, code as Z63.7 Other stressful life events affecting family and household.*
V61.20	Parent-Child Relational Problem	←		*No directly corresponding category, code as Z63.8 Other specified problems related to primary support group.*
V61.10	Partner Relational Problem	←→	Z63.0	Problems in relationship with spouse or partner
V61.8	Sibling Relational Problem	←→	F93.3	Sibling rivalry disorder
V62.81	Relational Problem NOS	←→	Z63.9	Problems related to primary support group, unspecified
Problems Related to Abuse or Neglect				
V61.21 / 995.54	Physical Abuse of Child, Focus of clinical attention on the perpetrator / Focus of clinical attention on the victim	←→ No corresponding differentiation in the ICD-10.	T74.1	Physical Abuse
V61.21 / 995.53	Sexual Abuse of Child, Focus of clinical attention on the perpetrator / Focus of clinical attention on the victim	←→ No corresponding differentiation in the ICD-10.	T74.2	Sexual Abuse
V61.21 / 995.52	Neglect of Child, Focus of clinical attention on the perpetrator / Focus of clinical attention on the victim	←→ No corresponding differentiation in the ICD-10.	T74.0	Neglect
V61.12 / V62.83 / 995.83	Physical Abuse of Adult By partner, focus of clinical attention on perpetrator / By other person, focus of clinical attention on perpetrator / Focus of clinical attention on the victim	←→ No corresponding differentiation in the ICD-10.	T74.1	Physical Abuse
V61.12 / V62.83 / 995.83	Sexual Abuse of Adult By partner, focus of clinical attention on perpetrator / By other person, focus of clinical attention on perpetrator / Focus of clinical attention on the victim	←→ No corresponding differentiation in the ICD-10.	T74.2	Sexual Abuse

	DSM-IV-TR	cross-walk		ICD-10
	Further Clinically Relevant Problems			
V15.81	Noncompliance With Treatment	←——→	Z91.1	Personal history of noncompliance with medical treatment and regimen
V65.2	Malingering	←——→	Z76.5	Malingerer (conscious simulation)
V71.01	Adult Antisocial Behavior	←—		*No directly corresponding category, code as Z72.8 Other problems related to lifestyle.*
V71.02	Child or Adolescent Antisocial Behavior	←—		*No directly corresponding category, code as Z72.8 Other problems related to lifestyle.*
V62.89	Borderline Intellectual Functioning	←—		*No directly corresponding category, code as R41.8 Other and unspecified symptoms and signs involving cognitive functions and awareness.*
780.9	Age-Related Cognitive Decline	←—		
V62.82	Bereavement	←—		*No directly corresponding category, consider F43.2 Adjustment disorder otherwise code as Z63.4 Disappearance and death of family member.*
V62.3	Academic Problem	←—		*No corresponding category. For V62.3 consider also F81.9 Developmental disorder of scholastic skills, unspecified. Otherwise code as Z65 Problems related to other psychosocial circumstances.*
V62.2	Occupational Problem	←—		
313.82	Identity Problem	←—		*No directly corresponding category. In childhood and adolescence code as F93.8 Other childhood emotional disorder.*
V62.89	Religious or Spiritual Problem	←—		*No directly corresponding category, code as Z71 Person encountering health services for other counselling and medical advice, not elsewhere classified.*
V62.4	Acculturation Problem	←——→	Z60.3	Acculturation difficulty
V62.89	Phase of Life Problem	←—		*No directly corresponding category, code as Z60.0 Problems of adjustment to life-cycle transitions.*
300.9	Unspecified Mental Disorder (nonpsychotic)	←——→	F99	Mental disorder, not otherwise specified
V71.09	No Diagnosis or Condition on Axis I	←—		*No corresponding category, code as Z03.2 Observation for suspected mental and behavioral disorder.*
799.9	Diagnosis or Condition Deferred on Axis I	←—		*No corresponding category, code as R69 Diagnosis deferred*
V71.09	No Diagnosis on Axis II	←—		*No corresponding category, code as Z03.2 Observation for suspected mental and behavioral disorder.*
799.9	Diagnosis Deferred on Axis II	←—		*No corresponding category, code as R46.8 Other symptoms and signs involving appearance and behavior.*

References

American Psychiatric Association (2000): Diagnostic and Statistical Manual of Mental Disorders (Fourth edition) (DSM-IV-TR). APA, Washington, DC

Bertelsen A (1999): Refections on the Clinical Utility of the ICD-10 and DSM-IV Classifications and their Diagnostic Criteria. Aust N Z J Psychiatry 33: 166-173

Cooper JE (1988): The Structure and Presentation of Contemporary Psychiatric Classifications as an International Perspective. Br J Psychiat 152: Supplement 1, 21-28

Cooper JE (1991): ICD-10 Classification of Mental and Behavioural Disorders with Glossary and Diagnostic Criteria for Research ICD-10: DCR-10. Churchill Livingstone, Edinburgh

Dilling H (1998): The Future of Diagnosis in Psychiatry. Fortschr Neurol Psychiatr 66: 36-42

Dilling H, Schulte-Markwort E, Freyberger HJ (1994a): Von der ICD-9 zur ICD-10. [*From ICD-9 to ICD-10*]. Huber, Bern

Dilling H, Mombour W, Schmidt MH, Schulte-Markwort E (Eds.) (1994b): Internationale Klassifikation psychischer Störungen. ICD-10 Kapitel V (F). Forschungskriterien. [*International Classification of Mental Disorders. ICD-10 Chapter V (F). Criteria for Research*]. Huber, Bern

Dilling H, Freyberger HJ (1999): Taschenführer zur Klassifikation psychischer Störungen. [*Pocket Guide to the Classification of Mental Disorders*]. Huber, Bern

Dilling H, Mombour W, Schmidt MH (Eds.) (1999): Internationale Klassifikation psychischer Störungen. ICD-10 Kapitel V (F). Klinisch-diagnostische Leitlinien. 3. Auflage. [*International Classification of Mental Disorders. ICD-10 Chapter V (F). Clinical Descriptions and Diagnostic Guidelines. Third edition*]. Huber, Bern

DIMDI (Ed.) (1994): Internationale statistische Klassifikation der Krankheiten und verwandter Gesundheitsprobleme. 10 Revision. ICD-10. Version 1.0. [*International Statistical Classification of Diseases and Related Health Problems. 10 Revision. ICD-10. Version 1.0.*]. Huber, Bern

Freyberger HJ, Schulte-Markwort E, Dilling H (1993a): Referenztabellen der WHO zum Kapitel V (F) der 10. Revision der Internationalen Klassifikation der Krankheiten (ICD-10): ICD-9 vs. ICD-10. [*WHO Reference Tables for Chapter V (F) of the 10th Revision of the International Classification of Diseases (ICD-10): ICD-9 vs. ICD-10*]. Fortschr Neurol Psychiatr 61: 109-127

Freyberger HJ, Schulte-Markwort E, Dilling H (1993b): Referenztabellen der WHO zum Kapitel V (F) der 10. Revision der Internationalen Klassifikation der Krankheiten (ICD-10): ICD-9 vs. ICD-10. [*WHO Reference Tables for Chapter V (F) of the 10th Revision of the International Classification of Diseases (ICD-10): ICD-9 vs. ICD-10*]. Fortschr Neurol Psychiatr 61: 128-143

Jablensky A (1999): The Nature of Psychiatric Classification: Issues beyond ICD-10 and DSM-IV. Aust N Z J Psychiatry 33: 137-144

Kendell RE (1991): Relationship between the DSM-IV and the ICD-10. J Abnorm Psychol 100: 297-301

Remschmidt H, Schmidt MH (1994): Multiaxiales Klassifikationsschema für psychische Störungen des Kindes- und Jugendalters nach ICD-10 der WHO. 3 rev. Auflage. [*Multiaxial Classification of Mental Disorders in Childhood and Adolescence in Accordance with ICD-10 of the WHO. Third revised edition*]. Huber, Bern

Saß H, Wittchen HU, Zaudig M (1996): Diagnostisches und Statistisches Manual Psychischer Störungen DSM-IV. [*Diagnostic und Statistical Manual of Mental Disorders DSM-IV*]. Hogrefe, Bern

Thompson JW, Pincus H (1989): A Crosswalk from DSM-III-R to ICD-10-CM. Am J Psychiatry 146: 1315-1319

Van Drimmelen-Krabbe J, Bertelsen A, Pull CH (1999): Ähnlichkeiten und Unterschiede zwischen ICD-10 und DSM-IV. [*Similarities and Differences between ICD-10 und DSM-IV*]. In: Helmchen H, Henn F, Lauter H, Sartorius N (Hrsg.): Psychiatrie der Gegenwart. 4. Auflage. Band II: Allgemeine Psychiatrie. [*Present Psychiatry. Fourth edition. Volume II: General Psychiatry*]. Springer, Heidelberg / New York

World Health Organization (1992): Classification of Mental and Behavioral Disorders – Clinical Descriptions and Diagnostic Guidelines. WHO, Geneva

World Health Organization (1993): Classification of Mental and Behavioral Disorders – Diagnostic Criteria for Research. WHO, Geneva